Endorsements

"If there's one thing we need in today's world, it's POSITIVITY. There's no shortage of it in Nick Kundrat's writing. His sense of humor and down-to-earth approach sets a great tone for thriving with diabetes."

—Gary Scheiner MS, CDE
Owner and Clinical Director, Integrated Diabetes Services
Author of *Think Like A Pancreas*
2014 Diabetes Educator of the Year

"This book is the in-depth reminder we all need that we're not alone in the daily challenges of T1D, combined with tons of real-life knowledge and tips. A must-read for anyone looking to improve how they think and *do* type 1 diabetes."

—Ginger Vieira
Author of Dealing with Diabetes Burnout and
Pregnancy with Type 1 Diabetes

"This book is fabulous! Nick puts the spotlight on the MANY admirable traits that those of living daily with type 1 share. This book provides a needed and much healthier perspective than thoughts of fear and pity that are too often portrayed. I've had T1D for 40 years, and my professional career is dedicated solely to helping others with T1D. I had tears in my eyes when I read this book. All of us with T1D need to be lifted up and feel proud of ourselves for living with T1D. This book does just that."

—Dr. Jody Stanislaw
Type 1 Diabetes Specialist
Virtual telemedicine practitioner
T1D x 40 years
www.drjodynd.com

POSITIVELY TYPE 1

"How a chronic illness can be your strongest motivator for an extraordinary life"

NICK KUNDRAT

Positively Type 1
by Nick Kundrat

Published by OS Press - Fuquay-Varina, NC

ISBN: 978-1-64184-354-6 (Hardcover)
ISBN: 978-1-64184-355-3 (Paperback)
ISBN: 978-1-64184-356-0 (Ebook)

Front Cover Design: Carly E. Baumgartner (Diabetic Design Co.)
@carly.with.diabetes

Thank you to JETLAUNCH.net for editing and book design.

Dedication

This is dedicated to all the amazing young type 1 warriors who I had the chance to interview for this book. Your lives are so much more than to be defined by a "disability." You are capable of so much and will accomplish amazing things. You weren't cursed with this disease—you were gifted with it—so use it wisely.

Acknowledgments

I can't thank everyone enough who was involved with this project. Special thanks to my fellow inspirational T1D's Dr. Jody Stanislaw, Ginger Vieira, and Gary Scheiner for their help and direction. To Dr. Reiner for his patience and care over the years. To Flora for giving me the means to both learn and educate. To John and Jeff for cultivating the communities that have energized me and so many others. For Camp Possibilities and Diabetes DESTINY for introducing me to the most amazing individuals I'll ever meet. To the parents of type 1s for raising such incredibly resilient children. To my parents for their love, support, and the intense "behind the scenes" work that comes along with having a child with T1D. To Meg for her early motivation and authorly experience. To Haley for her passion towards helping others with this condition. To Carly for her amazing artistic ability and constant encouragement. To Clyde and Dr. J for their entrepreneurial guidance. To God for his constant grace and blessings. To Original Strength for sparking my love of movement and education. To OS Press for being the ones to truly make this a reality and put in the countless hours to turn my idea into a publication. From the type 1 warriors who inspired it, to the friends and family who raised funds, to my amazing mentors who have helped to guide me along the way—I couldn't have done it without every one of you. Thank you.

Foreword

I hate diabetics. That should sound very strange, especially coming from someone who has devoted his entire career to dealing with diabetes. What I mean is that I hate the term "diabetic." When one says that Billy or Susan is a diabetic, they are telling you that Billy or Susan is defined by their diabetes and that they are unable to look at Billy or Susan without the word "diabetes" popping into their brain.

That is not the way it should be, and thankfully, that is not the way it is. Like other children, adolescents and adults, Billy and Susan are unique and special, one of a kind. They are not defined by their diabetes; they are defined by their hopes, dreams, deeds, and accomplishments. And they just happen to have diabetes.

It is especially gratifying to have observed over the years how many of my patients, instead of having diabetes define them, have, on their own terms, defined and embraced their diabetes. My patients have become teachers, accountants, attorneys, politicians, nurses, doctors, scientists, actors, and film producers, among others. Some, like the author, have traveled extensively. Many have been motivated to improve their health by engaging in physical activity and ended up excelling in sports well beyond what they might have accomplished had they not had diabetes. Others have been motivated by their diabetes to enter the fields of healthcare, medical research, or medical technology and make a difference to society in that manner.

Most of my patients take really good care of their diabetes (shout out to the author!), and many have used their diabetes as an additional motivational factor to go much further in life than they might have otherwise. For some, there is a silver lining to having diabetes, and a few, like the author, have turned their diabetes into something they are proud of and thankful for. As they say it, what they have become is not *despite* their diabetes, but *because of* their diabetes.

My hope, dear readers, is that you will gain a sense of inspiration and optimism from Nick and all the other wonderful type 1 warrior stories and use that to overcome and grow from any hurdles that you encounter on the challenging and beautiful hike on life's path.

—Barry J Reiner, MD

"The people who do really well when undergoing a personal disaster are those who look at the problem as an opportunity for change and not as a threat."

John Francis PhD from Planetwalker

Table of Contents

The Diagnosis

The year was 2002, and I was your typical four-year-old, doing typical four-year-old things: climbing trees, watching cartoons, being a mess, and living a life full of fun. No responsibility or care in the world. Life was good. Until, one day, my whole world changed.

I had come down with some kind of sickness. I was nauseated, thirsty, exhausted, and my parents were worried. To make their baby feel better, they looked to the pediatrician for answers. What he recommended worried them even more, a trip to the emergency room. For a stomach bug? No way was anything that seriously wrong—or so they thought. Per the doctor's wishes, we ended up in a crowded ER. After a long and stressful wait, the nurses ran some tests, and the results were shocking. I was diagnosed with type 1 diabetes.

Questions filled my head as nurses tried to teach me how to tackle my new "normal." What does this mean? Why is this happening to me? Is this my fault? Is this my parent's fault? Will I ever be normal? Can I ever eat sugar again? At age four, you don't understand much of anything, let alone the complexities of an auto-immune disease. My parents and I were terrified for my life ahead.

The way I lived my everyday life was about to change. Every single aspect of my life would have to be centered around diabetes. It never goes away, and I would never get a break from it. A simple family meal turned into measuring every morsel of food, checking my blood sugar, and giving myself insulin shots. Playing outside with my friends all day turned into having to take breaks inside treating low blood sugar levels. Every treatment decision I made had the power to either kill me or make me extremely ill. This was no joke. From that point on, I began my new life with the label of "diabetic," along with all the positives and negatives associated with it.

What is Diabetes?

Diabetes. Diabeetus. Whatever you've heard it called, chances are you've seen more about type 2 diabetes than type 1. They often get mixed up yet are extremely different conditions. Let me lay down some quick facts for you.

Type 1 diabetes (T1D) is an auto-immune disease, which means that our bodies are "attacking themselves" on the inside. In a person without diabetes, special cells called "beta cells" inside the pancreas create insulin, which is a hormone. Hormone is just a fancy word for a messenger, and insulin's job as a messenger is to signal our body when to lower the amount of sugar in our blood. It does this by taking the sugars from our bloodstream and sending it into our cells, which our cells use as fuel to keep our bodies working and give us energy.

When we eat, our blood sugar rises, so insulin helps to keep that in check and prevent it from rising too high. In someone with type 1, the body sees those beta cells that I mentioned earlier as the bad guy and destroys them. This could happen for a variety of uncontrollable reasons, usually genetic or environmental. It is not caused by being "fat" or unhealthy eating. You can be in your peak fitness and still be diagnosed with T1D. All this means is that our body has no signal to help lower the amount of sugar in our blood, so it can get much too high, causing some serious issues.

Another important hormone (messenger) called glucagon does the opposite of insulin, it signals the body to increase the amount of sugar in our blood. It does this by telling our liver to create (or release) more sugar, which then moves into our blood, where it can be sent all around the body. The creation of glucagon is also affected in people with T1D. When the amount of sugar in our blood goes below normal, the body cannot bring it back up on its own, putting us at risk of scary complications.

To break it down as simply as possible, all this confusing science-talk means that our bodies cannot properly balance the amount of sugar in the blood, so we must control it ourselves. It all comes down to controlling blood glucose levels. Glucose is just another fancy word for sugar, which comes from the food we eat. But why is our blood glucose level so important? Glucose is a very important source of fuel for many different parts of our body. It helps our brains stay sharp, our muscles keep pumping, and our energy levels stay high. It can also be harmful when we have too much or too little in our blood. Having good blood sugar levels can make all the difference.

In a non-diabetic human being, the target range of glucose in the blood fluctuates between roughly 80 to 120 mg/dL. Until you've lived with diabetes, it's hard to appreciate the fact that being within that range makes all the difference in how you feel, act, and perform in life. To further clarify, dropping too far below 80 mg/dL typically leaves ones shaky, tired, dizzy, and with barely enough energy to stand up. I often compare it to that run-down feeling you may get when you haven't eaten in a long time. Rising too far above 250 mg/dL can lead to nausea, increased thirst, headaches, and vomiting. Maintaining that range requires an intensive treatment consisting of insulin injections, exercise, food, and monitoring blood sugar levels. These injections can be done with syringes, prefilled insulin pens, or an insulin pump. The pump is that pager looking thing with the tube coming out of it that you may have seen people wearing. Monitoring blood glucose levels can be done by pricking your fingers and collecting a small blood sample or by a continuous glucose monitor (CGM). A CGM is a small patch that is worn on the skin and constantly tracks your blood glucose levels and transmits them to an app on your phone. Pretty cool, huh? Diabetes technology has come a long way, and it will only keep improving.

The ups and downs of living with diabetes are numerous, whether that's specifically related to blood glucose or just life in general. Every day is a balancing act, walking on the tightrope of blood sugar control. Falling off the tightrope one way, leading to blood sugar levels that are too high, can lead to intense sickness. The other way, low blood sugar levels can lead to unconsciousness and even a coma. Whether you live with T1D or know someone who does, you can appreciate how intense of a job it is taking care of your diabetes every day of every year of your entire life. In our world today, it's hard enough to maintain good health without diabetes, doing so while battling this condition takes true strength.

What affects blood sugar levels?

Controlling your blood sugar levels can't be too hard, right? Just don't eat a bunch of sweets and you'll be fine. Unfortunately, it's not that easy. There are a million things that affect blood sugar. Every little thing you eat, your activities, and so much more have an immense effect on your glucose levels. Here's a brief list of some of the most important ones, just to give you an idea of how difficult it can be:

Carbohydrate quantity: The more carbs you eat, the more your blood sugar will increase.

Carbohydrate type: Complex carbs (grains, for example) usually supply a slower, more steady increase in blood glucose, whereas simple carbs (a cookie or cake, for example) will create a sharp increase in blood glucose.

Other nutrients: Carbs aren't the only culprit in affecting blood glucose levels. Fat and protein intake can have its own hand in increasing your levels, usually kicking in later, rather than right after a meal/snack.

Other food factors: Caffeine, alcohol, dehydration, and even the timing of your meals can have major impacts on how you control your blood glucose, and they affect everyone differently.

Medication (insulin): This is the big one. How you dose your insulin has the greatest effect on your blood glucose levels because your body doesn't make it on its own. The amount of insulin, when you inject your insulin, and where on your body you inject your insulin affect your levels.

Activity levels: Depending on the type of exercise, your blood glucose levels can be sent in all different directions. Aerobic exercise like running or cycling will almost always drop your blood glucose low because your body is using up all that stored glucose for fuel for your muscles. Strength training like weight-lifting can either lower blood glucose (for the same reason as before) or raise it because your body is under more intense physical stress, so it thinks it needs to release more glucose to cope. Where you do your exercise (weather, temperature), the time of day you do your exercise, and when you exercise compared to what time you eat your meals can also have a big effect on your levels.

Stress levels: Usually, the more stress your body is under, the higher your blood sugar levels will be. This stress can be from school, work, lack of sleep, illness, and so much more. (Don't forget about the stress of dealing with diabetes itself!) Nowadays, it seems like everyone's pretty stressed all the time, so imagine having type 1 and having to cope with all these different stressors and taking care of your blood sugar levels at the same time.

Random factors: Something as simple as getting a sunburn can cause your blood sugars to be higher than normal. Being at a higher altitude than normal can raise or drop your levels. For girls, being on their monthly cycle can drastically change blood sugar levels. Seasonal allergies can also raise your sugar levels.

Every little thing affects blood sugar levels.

These are just a few big examples, but there's so many more. Hopefully, this gives you a bit more of an appreciation for what it's really like trying to keep those numbers in check.

No Walk in the Park

Allow me to do another quick breakdown of a confusing science topic known as the natural history of disease. This is essentially explaining the process of how we, as humans, obtain and fight a disease. It begins with being free of symptoms (meaning you're perfectly healthy), then you obtain the disease, typically through genetic or environmental factors. Now that you have the disease, next comes the treatment (dealing with your disease with medical or lifestyle interventions), and circles back around to being free of symptoms. In other words, you contract a disease, you treat that disease, and you get back to normal life as you were. With type 1 diabetes, it's not that simple. Type 1 diabetes is unique in that it's what's called a chronic condition. Chronic means it lasts a long time, and for T1D specifically, it lasts our entire lives.

The story of type 1 starts like any other disease; being free of symptoms, then you obtain the disease, then move on to treatment—but it ends at treatment. With type 1, the treatment allows for survival, but will not return you back to symptom freedom as with most other diseases. You'll now find your new normal for the rest of your life in this realm of treatment, along with all the successes and failures that come along with it. Because of this, diabetes can take a massive toll on your health and well-being. We take care of our condition 24 hours a day, 7 days a week. We never get time off; we never get a break. It takes an insane amount of work every day just to take care of your diabetes. Think about all that, in addition to everything else in your day that is not diabetes-related. It's nothing short of overwhelming, both mentally and physically.

Now, believe me, I get that this is a scary thought and one that I wrestled with a lot throughout my life. But don't let that fill you with fear. Let that excite you for the new you that is to come. Think of it as a bit of a rebirth, as cheesy as that might sound. Hopefully, by the end of this book, you'll have forgotten about those negative things that come along with T1D and be pumped for the amazing new super-you that wouldn't have been possible without your diagnosis.

Speaking of scary thoughts, mental health issues are more common in our society today than they ever have been, and even more so for us living with type 1. Think about it like this, at whatever age you were diagnosed, you started a full-time job. Most eight-year-olds I know don't have full-time jobs, but with diabetes, that's unfortunately the case. No wonder everyone's tired and overwhelmed. According to the *Canadian Journal of Medicine*, young adults and children with type 1 are at significantly higher risk of anxiety, depression, and suicide than their non-diabetic counterparts.

This all particularly hit home for me the summer of 2019 at diabetes camp. I was volunteering as a counselor and part of camp this year was circle discussions about "diabetes burnout." If you aren't familiar with the term, diabetes burnout refers to the negative emotions and burdens of self-management related to living with diabetes. This can present itself as anger toward your diagnosis, feeling controlled by your diabetes, or feeling alone or isolated and even avoiding your diabetes management overall (Robinson 2020). This can obviously be extremely harmful to our health and lead to some pretty nasty issues.

As we went around the circle, kids told heart-wrenching stories about their own mental health struggles when it comes to their diabetes. This left everyone teary-eyed, me included. But at the same time, it made me realize something that has ended up guiding my life since and inspired the book you're reading right now.

The Big Realization

Listening to these stories, I honestly couldn't quite relate. I was extremely empathetic to what everyone had gone through, but I hadn't experienced anything similar myself. Though diabetes hasn't been a walk in the park, I would never say I struggled with diabetes burnout at all. If anything, I've experienced the complete opposite.

My entire life, I've had it within me to see everything through a positive lens. It was imparted to me early on that with type 1, my situation would not change. What did that mean? My attitude had to change. Rather than seeing my condition as a burden to carry with me for the rest of my life, I used it as my most powerful motivator. I saw it as the biggest challenge I would ever face, and we all know what comes from overcoming big challenges—even bigger successes. As odd as it sounds, type 1 has been the greatest gift I've ever received. While it's indeed a life-threatening disease, it has also been a strong force, pushing me toward excellence in life.

With my own experience, and after years of work in camps and hospitals with kids with type 1, it's easy to see that they are a pretty remarkable bunch of little humans. Whether they are athletes, musicians, students, actors, dancers, sons, daughters, sisters, brothers, friends, or anything in between, they are some of the strongest, most resilient people I've had the pleasure of meeting. Despite all the insensitive questions, weird looks, and constant judgment from others, they continue to wade through life with bright smiles and kind hearts.

This also made me realize that the way we educate young people with type 1 is a bit backward. We only focus on the things they'll lose in life, such as how they won't have the freedom that most kids have, how they won't always get to eat exactly what they want, or how they'll be forced to inject themselves with insulin. While this may be true and important to learn, we're missing out on half of the information. We conveniently miss all the amazing things they'll gain from living with diabetes, like the amazing skills they'll master, the character traits they'll build, and the tight-knit communities and relationships they'll cultivate.

Just like anything in life, balance is important. I'm not voting that we stop educating kids with type 1 how to properly inject their insulin. What I am pushing for is a perspective shift in the way we look at life with diabetes or any chronic illness. The similar struggles we all go through can be seen as challenges to conquer instead of burdens to carry. Diabetes has the power to give you so many amazing things that make you who you are and who you will become. I want to share those with you in detail to hopefully inspire, motivate, and open your eyes to all the amazing benefits of living with type 1 diabetes.

Toughness

\ ˈtəf \ : *capable of enduring strain, hardship, or severe labor : characterized by severity or uncompromising determination (Merriam-Webster 2020)*

What comes to mind when you hear the word "tough?" For many of us, it triggers thoughts of football players, motorcycle riders, and MMA fighters. But why doesn't anyone mention the kids who haven't even finished primary school who spend countless hours every week administering insulin shots all over their bodies? Sounds pretty tough to me.

As you can probably tell, life with type 1 diabetes is no walk in the park. It's a constant daily battle. This is nothing to get down about, though. Enduring this fight constantly will help you to become extremely tough and resilient with your diabetes and wherever else life takes you. I like to compare it to how gymnasts' hands get thick and calloused after spending lots of time working on the rings and the bars. That's kind of like us. We go through some tough stuff every day, which helps us to build up mentally and physically to be rugged and sturdy.

However, that doesn't mean it won't come with hardships along the way. Flashback to 2010, I was twelve years old and scared to death of inserting my own insulin pump. My parents had been doing it for me since I was six years old, but I couldn't muster up the courage to do it myself. It took lots of tears and yelling, but one day, I just decided to go for it. I specifically remember saying to my parents afterward, "Wow, that wasn't bad at all," and I've been doing it ever since. It's moments like these that build us type 1s up to be strong, tough, and resilient.

I've been injected with needles and devices for essentially my entire life, so now anything medically related doesn't even phase me. While some may wince in pain or even faint during a blood draw, I'm able to chat with the nurse about how her day is going as if there weren't a two-inch needle flopping out of my arm.

There's no doubt that kids with type 1 face adversity every time they step outside. It could be because they must spend time in the nurse's office and miss class or because there are some mean kids making fun of them for a disease they don't even understand. Some days can be exhausting, both physically and emotionally. While this may seem to tear you down in the moment, you'll look back later and see how much stronger it truly made you. All these struggles are just mini-challenges where you'll walk in scared and confused but walk out with a layer of toughness unlike any other group of people.

Spotlight: Maura C.

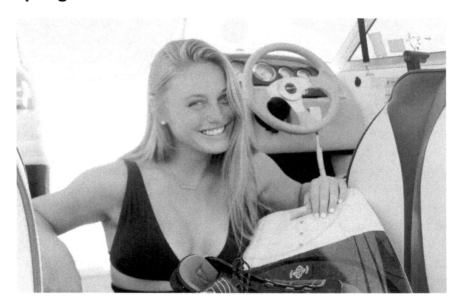

Bio

Maura is twenty years old and was diagnosed with type 1 at age seven. She loves being outdoors, whether that's on a boat, off-roading, or hiking. Maura also plays division 1 lacrosse at Arizona State University—in other words: she is pretty awesome. Maura is one of my closest friends with type 1, always has a smile on her face, and is an absolute blast to be around.

How has diabetes positively impacted your life?

I think diabetes has probably impacted my life in more positive ways than I would like to admit. First, it taught me that anything is possible and that having a chronic illness does not have to slow you down or keep you from following your dreams. It has positively changed my mindset when it comes to a lot of things.

If you could tell someone newly diagnosed something you've learned living with T1, what would it be?

When I first got diagnosed, all my doctors were telling me were the things that I wasn't going to be able to do, how I was not going to be able to play sports, have sleepovers, eat what I wanted, etc. They were wrong. I would tell newly diagnosed people that you can do absolutely everything any other person can do. Yes, sometimes it might be harder, and there are going to be obstacles you will have to overcome, but you can do it. Everyone expects you to fail or give up. They don't expect you to rise up and defy the odds, so defy them. The people who were in my life when I was diagnosed would never have thought in a million years that I would be living my dream of playing a division one sport, but here I am. Yes, some days are definitely harder than others, but when those days happen, I just remind myself of every other bad day I went through to get to where I am, and that I got through it. Everything I do is ten times more rewarding because I am doing it while managing a chronic illness. Do not let diabetes control your life—you take control. Don't let diabetes define who you are.

How has type 1 given you toughness? Please explain a specific story.

Diabetes has given me true toughness. I don't believe that one specific story defines why I find this to be true, but a multitude of experiences do. Every time I have had what I call a "bad diabetes day," I have found the strength to continue on and get done what I need to get done. I have persevered through the highs and the lows, literally, to get where I am. No matter what diabetes did to try to hold me back, I never let it.

A certain set of experiences that come to mind happened during my first semester of college. We were practicing six days a week, and I could not seem to get my blood sugar levels under control, I would go low, then go high, then bolus for the high and plummet again. It was frustrating because not only did it make me feel very sick, but it was affecting my performance at practice. No matter what I did, nothing seemed to be working, yet I never gave up. I kept trying new things, and there was a lot of trial and error. Eventually, things started to work, my blood sugar levels were under control, and my performance was better because I physically felt better. Looking back, if I had given up and never found a solution, I probably would not be on my team, and the dream I worked so hard for would have vanished. Diabetes has made me tougher, and that is a trait I will carry with me for the rest of my life and apply to every challenge that comes my way.

Empathy

em·pa·thy | \ ˈem-pə-thē \ : *the action of understanding, being aware of, being sensitive to, and vicariously experiencing the feelings, thoughts, and experience of another of either the past or present without having the feelings, thoughts, and experience fully communicated in an objectively explicit manner (Merriam-Webster 2020)*

Living with a chronic illness like type 1 builds strong character and gives one true respect for how delicate life really is. A life filled with daily struggles allows for a special appreciation of the joys and wonders that our time on earth can offer. The many individuals I know who are battling type 1 are some of the most empathetic human beings I've met. They radiate kindness and understanding regarding the troubles that they and others have faced.

Despite the many positives, life with diabetes is full of rough patches. Whether those are dangerously low blood sugar, high blood sugar, missed doses, pump site failures, or other frustrating difficulties, we are plagued with challenges daily. This means that, as a person with type 1, you learn to tackle the tough days and embrace the good ones. This mindset allows us to find the calm during the storm and help others do the same. Type 1 is a hidden condition meaning that, unless you see someone giving their insulin shots, you could never tell that they have diabetes. The fact that lots of our struggles go on behind the scenes, we are able to understand others who also face hidden obstacles, whether that be disease, social struggles, mental health issues, or anything else.

I don't know one human being who doesn't go through struggles in life. At some point or another, we've all been faced with something to battle through. But remember, life is so good! This is exactly why empathy is an overwhelmingly important skill to have. Type 1 teaches us to look past those tough times, appreciate life, and help everyone around us do the same. The wonderful people I know who battle type 1 have an uncanny ability to understand and relate to others' struggles, spreading positivity and love everywhere life takes them.

Spotlight: Ben S.

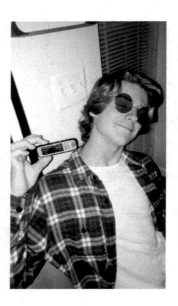

Bio

Ben, better known as "Beano" is seventeen years old and was diagnosed with diabetes at age five. He's an outgoing guy with some of the best dance moves I've ever seen. He loves rock music and enjoys going to concerts and hanging out with his buddies. Ben runs track and cross-country at his school and plays guitar at home, with friends, and in his school ensemble. He also loves working with his hands and making art. One of his favorite classes in school is 3D Design, where he gets to craft cool sculptures, vases, cups, and more. He's an adventurous dude who loves going on road trips and adventures with his friends, seeing new cities and exploring.

How has diabetes positively impacted your life?

Diabetes has made me more mindful of my body and conscious of my health. I feel like it's made me tougher because I've had to overcome challenges that not everybody has to face. It's helped me gain discipline, which has carried over into my academics and athletic career. Also, I think it helped me become more mature and responsible.

If you could tell someone newly diagnosed something you've learned living with T1, what would it be?

You will have some bad diabetes days, that's inevitable. Sometimes, your numbers just don't cooperate, and it can ruin your mood or even ruin a whole day. My best advice is that your reaction is what matters. Try as hard as you can not to get discouraged. Find a way to vent your frustrations that works for you. For me, it's going on a run or blasting some angry music. Your numbers don't define you. Also, if you aren't truly impaired due to high or low blood sugar, never use diabetes as a cop-out or an excuse, even though it can be very tempting sometimes. Don't exploit it; be better than that. I can't tell you how many times I've wanted to blame a mistake I've made on diabetes when it was my own fault. People will admire you more for struggling and overcoming challenges while being humble.

How has type 1 given you empathy? Please explain a specific story.

Diabetes has made me more empathetic because I can relate to others who may be going through a struggle that isn't visible on the outside. This is the nature of diabetes, as you can't just look at someone and know that they have it. Because of my experience dealing with diabetes, I've had to learn to operate with a level head, even when I'm not feeling well physically. Often, when other people are going through unseen struggles, they also put on this false persona of being just fine. I know exactly how that feels and how frustrating it can be, and I'm able to understand and share those feelings. In practice, this means that I feel like I am less quick to jump to conclusions about why someone is acting a certain way rather than consider what they might be going through.

A certain time when I felt like my empathy really came through was a few weeks back on a drive with my friends Josh and Chris (whose names have been changed). My buddies and I love taking long night drives to random places just to listen to music and talk.

It's become a tradition for us. Something about being stuck in a car together just brings things out of people that you wouldn't normally talk about at school.

Recently, we'd all been discussing our plans for college, and everyone's plans were drastically different. My friend Chris wants to get out of his hometown and dive straight into big-city life. My other friend, Josh, who works as a lifeguard tirelessly, wants to stay in-state and feels constrained to one school due to his incredible fear of debt. For me, I'm unsure about everything, but I do want the college experience at a relatively cheap cost, and I'm still not fully convinced of even going to college because of my infatuation with the trades.

As Josh was explaining his views, Chris and I started questioning him a lot. We figured out was that Josh measures success entirely based on his monetary worth. Josh wants a high-paying career, and nothing gets him excited like making money. For me, this view on life was incredibly hard to understand, and frankly, it kind of frustrated me because it was so different from my own. I think that I measure success primarily based on how many awesome experiences I've had and how many deep bonds I've formed with people. I just want to be known as a well-traveled, wise, great-to-talk-to-no-matter-who-you-are kind of guy.

As we were discussing, I found it really hard to put myself in Josh's shoes. But as Josh went into more depth about his childhood and family life, I started to understand. After hearing everything about Josh and his story, I was able to put myself in his shoes, and it really made more sense why he was limiting himself to one school. I had to realize that, before you start getting frustrated at someone for the way they think, you have to try to understand what they're going through. Diabetes has helped me do just that.

Hardworking

hard·work·ing | \ ˈhärd-ˈwər-kiŋ \ : *constantly, regularly, or habitually engaged in earnest and energetic work : INDUSTRIOUS, DILIGENT (Merriam-Webster 2020)*

Living with type 1 creates individuals who must work diligently every day simply to stay alive. T1D involves intensive, constant treatment every hour of every day consisting of monitoring blood sugar levels, counting carbs, administering insulin, and so much more. How can this be a good thing? Well, hear me out.

For someone without T1D, sitting down to eat dinner is simple and not very exciting. Cook the food, eat, then clean up. It's a typical ritual that we all do daily. For someone with type 1, that simple act becomes amazingly complex. First, we must carefully measure all the ingredients going into the meal to ensure a proper carb count. Each ingredient is carefully calculated in measuring cups and spoons because the more exact the measurement, the easier it becomes to treat. After measuring, we cook the meal and put it on the plate. However, rather than chowing down, we must check our blood sugar level and use that number to judge how big of an insulin dose we need to cover the meal. This dose also depends on the number of carbohydrates in the meal and what type of carbs (complex and nutrient-dense or simple and calorie-dense), which determines our insulin needs. After the correct amount of insulin is decided, we must next actually give the insulin, whether that's through a shot or an insulin pump. After ten or fifteen minutes, we can finally eat, clear the table, and do the dishes, yet it doesn't end there. For the next few hours, we must keep a close watch on our blood sugars to make sure we gave the correct dose, and the meal didn't affect us in ways we didn't expect. Now think about this same process with every single meal or snack every day for the rest of your life.

I'm not sure about you, but to me, that sounds like a lot of hard work. A few days of that and you non-diabetic human beings would be exhausted. Yet, for us, it's not a choice. Not to get super serious on you, but we do this, or we die, plain and simple. We must work hard for all the simple things most people take for granted. But don't take this as complaining. Doing this for essentially my entire life has taught me how to work hard for everything in life, and the same goes for anyone living with T1D. Working hard to stay alive every day teaches us diligence in everything else we do. Whether it's school, work, or relationships, we're blessed with the ability to work hard and give our all in every situation.

Spotlight: Bailey G.

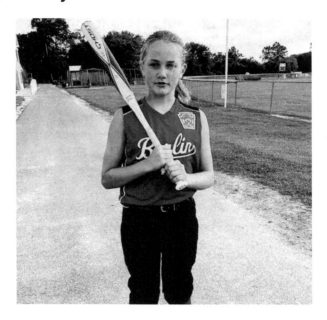

Bio

Bailey is twelve years old and was diagnosed with diabetes at age nine. She is an extremely talented athlete who plays softball, basketball, and field/indoor hockey. She and her team recently won the Little League softball state championship and had the chance to travel to Connecticut for the regional tournament. While Bailey was there, she got to tour ESPN headquarters and meet a sports anchor whom she really looks up to. Outside of sports, she loves the beach, drawing, and baking delicious desserts.

How has diabetes positively impacted your life?

Having diabetes has allowed me to go to diabetes camp where I have made new friends and learned that there are many other children just like me with type one diabetes. Diabetes has also made me want to be a role model for younger/newly diagnosed with T1D.

If you could tell someone newly diagnosed something you've learned living with T1, what would it be?

Diabetes may seem scary at first, but it will come easier soon and will make you a tougher person at the end.

How has type 1 made you hardworking? Please explain a specific story.

Being an athlete with type one diabetes means having to work hard, playing through the highs and lows of my blood sugar levels, and trying to avoid blood sugar rollercoasters during and after sports. I don't always want to stop playing to eat snacks or get insulin, but I know that I must so that I can stay in the game. In my Little League state championship, my blood sugar was going up fast. My mom wanted to give me insulin, but I wanted to get out on the field. But I stopped and allowed her to give me a shot because I knew that if I didn't, I might start feeling bad, and I didn't want to let my team down.

Motivation

mo·ti·va·tion | \ ˌmō-tə-ˈvā-shən \ : *the act or process of motivating*
: the condition of being motivated : a motivating force, stimulus, or
influence : INCENTIVE, DRIVE
(Merriam-Webster 2020)

For you, hearing the word "motivation" may elicit images of motivational speakers spreading their message on a huge stage. It may evoke thoughts of Instagram "fitness influencers" posting workout videos complete with hashtag #motivation #hardwork #nevergivein #inspiration and so on. In my (quite biased) opinion, life with type 1 creates motivated individuals unlike anything else. With the biggest incentive of all, your life, in your hands at all times, you must remain resilient throughout every single day.

With any activity in life, what you put in is what you get out. Take your job, for example. The harder you work, the higher you can climb within your company, leading to a higher paycheck. The same can be said for a parent. The more time and love you give to your child, the better they grow and flourish. With diabetes, the same reigns true. With your health on the line, the more careful you are with treatments like insulin dosing and carb counting, the better your long and short-term health can be. Diabetes left untreated can lead to rather disgusting health issues. I don't think anyone wants to lose their toes, feet, or eyesight, right? Keeping these possible issues in mind can be scary, yet even better, can be a strong incentive for always being careful with your treatment.

There are also a million and one factors that influence blood sugar levels, as you read earlier in this book, and you can only control a few of them. You begin to learn that with even the most motivated, hardworking type 1s, they have their off days where they just can't seem to control their blood sugar levels. Realizing that your health isn't always under your control is both humbling and terrifying. Yet, it can be one of the strongest factors that help to further the intense motivation to take charge of your own health and be your best self every single day.

Spotlight: Michael R.

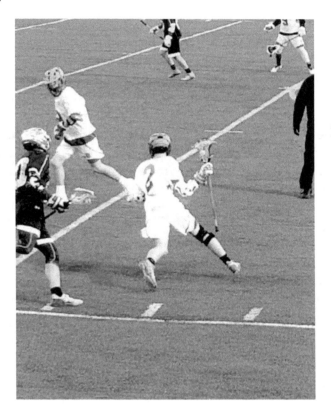

Bio

Mike is seventeen years old and was diagnosed with diabetes at age four. He is a high school student who plays lacrosse and soccer and runs track. He's one of the funniest and friendliest dudes I know. Mike may seem quiet at first, but you can always count on him to crack a killer joke with impeccable timing.

How has diabetes positively impacted your life?

Diabetes has helped give me a positive outlook on everything I do. It has also helped to keep me healthy with my diet, and most importantly, it has helped me meet some of the nicest people I know.

If you could tell someone newly diagnosed something you've learned living with T1, what would it be?

It can only stop you if you let it. You're just a normal kid with a little something special. It can't hurt you if you don't let it, and it won't negatively affect you if you take care of it.

How has type 1 given you motivation? Please explain a specific story.

Diabetes has given me motivation through all it's challenging times. I learn from these challenges, and I have realized it is the biggest obstacle in my life. Despite this, any other obstacle I face in life will not be as significant as diabetes. Throughout middle school, I was never really a good student. My grades weren't amazing, and I was generally never motivated. High school was when I finally realized nothing in my life is more challenging than diabetes. From that day, my GPA has been good, I have been excelling in lacrosse and other sports, I have been constantly motivated, and I always remind myself that I do a great job taking care of my biggest obstacle in life!

Problem-solving

*: the process or act of finding a solution to a problem
(Merriam–Webster 2020)*

often compare life with type 1 as one big puzzle that always has a few pieces missing. No matter how diligent one is with their treatment, there will always be things out of your control. As I mentioned before, this shouldn't be seen as a downer, rather a motivator to push you further.

This "diabetic puzzle" is a hefty one to tackle. With each separate piece being its own problem to solve, it can add up to a lot of time and energy being devoted to diabetes. Every blood test, every insulin shot, every measuring cup filled with food, every pump site change are all their own mini problems to solve. I've heard that on average, people with T1D make 180 more decisions per day than a person without diabetes! Mind. Blown.

Take an insulin shot, for example. You must count the number of carbs you plan to eat, calculate the appropriate dosage, decide where to inject, and decide when to inject. Imagine doing this multiple times every day. Another example would be treating low blood sugar levels. Let's say your blood sugar is dropping in the middle of your run. You must stop and calculate how many carbohydrates to eat to bring your sugar up to the correct level. Too many carbs, and your blood sugar goes too high, not enough, and your blood sugar drops lower and lower. Throughout all this, you begin to become pretty amazing at solving problems and thinking on your feet.

Living with type 1, we have been given a chance every day to build amazingly important life skills through our daily routines. Things that take others decades to learn, we master in a few short years. I know children with diabetes as young as seven years old who are better problem solvers than most adults will ever be. This is pretty remarkable as it creates individuals who can tackle almost anything life throws at them, with their diabetes as an afterthought.

Spotlight: Megan W.

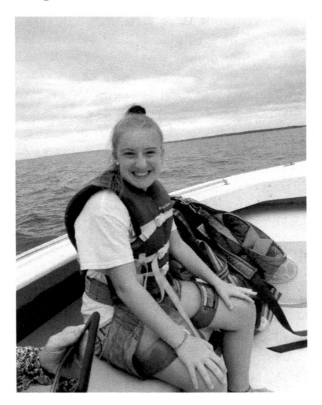

Bio

Megan is seventeen years old and was diagnosed with diabetes at age six. She's currently in school, has a job, and in her words, "can give a needle in a dark, moving car," which is quite impressive in my book. Megan's obviously talented, and she is always full of energy, bringing positivity everywhere she goes.

How has diabetes positively impacted your life?

I've matured fast and learned how to be responsible for myself and others. I can also do quick mental math in my head from all of the carb counting I do.

If you could tell someone newly diagnosed something you've learned living with T1, what would it be?

Don't expect everything to be easy, you can do everything right and still not get it right. It's not your fault, it's completely normal, so always keep your head up!

How has type 1 made you a good problem-solver? Please explain a specific story.

Diabetes has given me the skill of problem-solving through all the (literal) highs and lows. There have been many times over the years where I've had large ketones, with both highs and lows, and it's always a struggle to figure it out. Type 1 has given me the skills to find the causes of these seemingly unexplainable occurrences and has allowed me to do it with minimal stress.

Independence

in·de·pen·dence | \ ˌin-də-ˈpen-dən(t)s \ : *the quality or state of being independent (Merriam-Webster 2020)*

Living with type 1 is a task that nobody can truly handle on their own. Whether it's your mom checking your blood sugar in the middle of the night or your endocrinologist helping you figure out your insulin doses, it always takes a supportive team to reach your ideal health with diabetes. Battling a chronic illness teaches independence unlike anything else. That supportive team would fall apart without the independent young leader who's orchestrating the whole operation. I personally know young children with type 1 who exhibit far more independence than most college kids I know who live on their own.

Having your life in your hands every day builds strong self-determination. To put it in perspective, if you were to accidentally overdose the amount of insulin for a meal by not paying attention and just moving the syringe down a little bit further than it should've gone, you could be in a coma within an hour or two. Being only a few units off the correct dosage can wreak absolute havoc on your body. This is the ultimate incentive for taking good care of your diabetes and overall health.

The example I always love to share with people is how, when I was young, I would come home right after school and finish my homework without being told before playing outside. This may not sound like much, but any parents reading this know what I'm getting at. Think about most six-year-olds and the absolute nightmare it is trying to get them to do any sort of work, especially after school. I was independent, I knew what needed to be done, and I made sure I made it happen. I attribute this 100% to my early diagnosis of type 1. I learned from a young age that I was responsible for my own health and success; I always worked hard to make sure I did my absolute best with my treatment and every other part of life.

Learning the delicacy of your life at such an early age creates individuals who are great at taking care of their own health and are in touch with those around them at the same time. I've watched children as young as five years old drawing up lifesaving liquid medication from a vial into a syringe and injecting it into their skin all on their own without the slightest wince. If that doesn't exhibit real strength and independence, I don't know what does.

Spotlight: Abigail F.

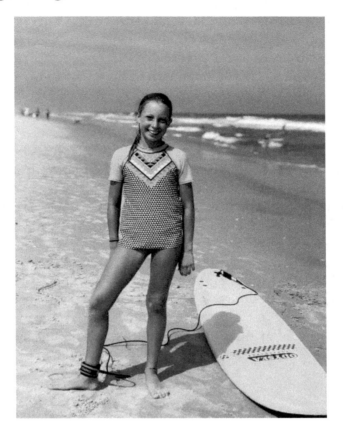

Bio

Abigail is twelve years old and was diagnosed with diabetes at age eight. Her all-time favorite activity is dance. Abigail has been dancing since age four and can tackle all kinds of different styles, including ballet, lyrical, pointe, tap, and jazz. (Ballet is her favorite.) She hopes to one day attend a ballet school, become a prima ballerina, and continue dancing as long as she can. Outside of dancing, she also participates in her local swim team, rides horses, and rides bikes with her brothers. Obviously, she doesn't let her diabetes get her down one bit.

How has diabetes positively impacted your life?

Diabetes has its ups and downs, but it has affected my life because, without my condition, I would have never had the awesome summer camp and friends I do now. The summer camp is called Camp Possibilities, and it has changed everyone's life who has gone to it. We get to sleep in a cabin of five or six kids and usually two counselors. It's really cool. What I love most about camp is their game of gaga ball. A lot of people there are obsessed with it, including me.

If you could tell someone newly diagnosed something you've learned living with T1, what would it be?

If I had to tell a newly diagnosed person something, I would say this quote, "Why stand in when you were made to stand out?" If people have a problem with you not doing something normal like other kids do because of your condition, kindly explain to them what it is you have and tell them you are fully capable of doing anything you desire. If someone says, "Oh, you ate too much junk food or sugar; that's what happened, right?", you probably want to get mad at them for even thinking that, but let's face it, they probably were never taught what Type 1 was. Instead, explain what it really is!

How has type 1 made you independent? Please explain a specific story.

One way that diabetes has made me independent is that, after a while, you must give yourself shots. My mom told me a while ago that if l wanted to do sleepovers with friends, then I would have to give myself shots. I couldn't have my mom at all my sleepovers! About ten months after I was diagnosed, my mom was going out to eat with the teachers at her work, and so that meant she wouldn't be there to give me my dinner shot. It was a hard decision I had to make whether my Mimi (my grandmother) would do it or if I would do it myself for the first time. I chose to do it myself, and after that, I don't let anyone, even trained nurses, give me my shots.

Responsibility

re·spon·si·bil·i·ty | \ ri-ˌspän(t)-sə-ˈbi-lə-tē \ : *the quality or state of being responsible: such as : moral, legal, or mental accountability : RELIABILITY, TRUSTWORTHINESS : something for which one is responsible : BURDEN (Merriam–Webster 2020)*

Individuals living with type 1 diabetes must exhibit responsibility unlike any other group of people. This disease forces us to grow up faster than our peers, which is a positive in my eyes. As I've mentioned, life with type 1 is a delicate balance between life and death, sickness and health. The more responsible you are with caring for yourself, the better your life can be in the present and future. The healthier you are right now, the healthier you can be as an adult, free of horrific complications that nobody wants to deal with.

Staying accountable for correct medication dosing, carb counting, and everything else isn't much of a choice for us. If we don't do it correctly and decide to slack off, we feel the consequences in our blood sugar levels, our mood, and our overall health. Even something as simple as being responsible for carrying around your own medications keeps you in check as you know the dangers that await if you leave your supplies behind. (But that's not to say that we all haven't forgotten our diabetes bags under the table at Chick-fil-A a few times.)

We are forced to be responsible since we were given this heavy weight to carry on our shoulders every day. However, the responsibility you build from living with type 1 applies to more than just your condition. All the children I've had the pleasure of meeting who live with type 1 are all extremely mature and responsible for their age. Most of them know more about the human body than most adults and can decipher confusing medical mumbo-jumbo like it's nothing. They also tend to be a leader among their friends, and given their grown-up demeanor, they can be relied on and trusted.

Through all this adult-like responsibility, one might think that your care-free childhood magic is lost, but I've never heard anyone with type 1 complain about missing out on their childhood due to their condition. They choose to cherish those easy-going times in their lives and remain humbled about the not-so-easy ones. This means that the good times of your life are further magnified for the amazing memories that they are. Rather than being held back by their condition, people with type 1 are pushed forward with a boldly optimistic outlook leading the way.

Spotlight: Zach S.

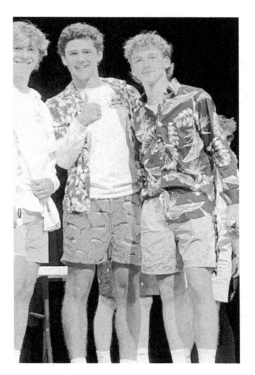

Bio

Zach is sixteen years old and was diagnosed with diabetes at age ten. He is a high school student and is one of the funniest kids I know. In school, Zach participates in soccer and lacrosse and is his class's vice president, along with an impressive #1 class rank (Go Friars!). Outside of school, he enjoys club soccer and is (slowly) learning to play the ukulele.

How has diabetes positively impacted your life?

Since being diagnosed, a lot of challenges that "normal" teens face has been much easier for me. Whether it be time-management skills with homework or making good decisions at parties because I know I must watch my number, diabetes has made me much more responsible. That added layer of responsibility since I was diagnosed seemed like a lot at the beginning but has helped a lot in the long run.

If you could tell someone newly diagnosed something you've learned living with T1, what would it be?

I would say that the hardest part is definitely the beginning. So many people think it's too much right off the bat and give up, which could be absolutely devastating for their health. There are always support systems around you (even if you don't know where to look), and if you keep your cool and stay focused all the time, it gets way easier.

How has type 1 made you responsible? Please explain a specific story.

Like I mentioned previously, diabetes has made me much more responsible. A great example of this is from homecoming at my school just a little while ago. After the dance, there were plenty of people making bad decisions at different parties and hangouts after a great night. A lot of those kids would go on to get in trouble with their parents or even with the police if they weren't careful. I knew that I shouldn't make these choices for multiple reasons, but by far the biggest reason was that I knew I had to pay attention to my glucose levels. Even with that added responsibility, I had a really fun night and stayed out of trouble afterward.

Composure

com·po·sure | \ kəm-ˈpō-zhər \ : *a calmness or repose especially of mind, bearing, or appearance: SELF-POSSESSION (Merriam-Webster 2020)*

In our world today, it's easy to get overwhelmed. Work, school, kids, parents, sports, health—there are millions of responsibilities to get buried under. Maintaining composure in our fast-paced world is tough, to say the least. Add type 1 diabetes into that equation, and it becomes next to impossible.

I can remember thousands of times in my life where I got angry at my diabetes. Whether it was a pump site that failed and stopped giving me insulin or a CGM that just wouldn't stay stuck to my skin, all those little challenges really tested my temper. There've been plenty of instances where I would've liked to throw in the towel and say goodbye to my diabetes altogether. Years and years of all these little annoyances have allowed me to become one of the calmest and even-tempered individuals I know. There isn't much that really bothers me anymore. I like to say that diabetes is like the person in the woods who pokes the bear repeatedly, and you are the bear. Get poked enough (no needle pun intended), and little things begin not to bother you too much anymore.

The same holds true for lots of my friends who've lived with type 1 for a while. I've seen firsthand many times when something goes wrong for one of them, they attack it with a "let's keep trying!" attitude. Type 1 allows you to realize that there's no reason to get mad at dumb little things in life that you can't control. Looking at life through this lens positively changes your mood every day and your outlook on life in general.

Living with diabetes, you also build insanely strong mental composure and are able to come across as calm and collected, even if you aren't. If you have type 1, you know all too well that there are always a million things happening in your head. What's my blood sugar level? Is there any juice around? Do I feel thirsty? How much insulin do I have left in my system? Is my insulin pump working right? Do I look pale? We're constantly surveying the environment, making sure our numbers are in range, and checking in with how our body is feeling among heaps of other things. This may sound like a lot, but believe it or not, this is the dialogue that goes on constantly in my head all day, every day. I could be up in front of my entire class, giving a presentation, clicking through a PowerPoint and answering questions, and still be thinking about my diabetes simultaneously.

This ability to stay cool, calm, collected, multitask with ease, and handle diabetes makes for some remarkable people capable of accomplishing amazing things.

Spotlight: Ashlyn B.

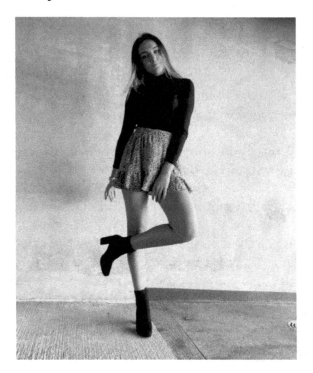

Bio

Ashlyn is nineteen years old and was diagnosed with diabetes at age eight. She loves to be active and hits the gym pretty much daily. She's also a beast on the volleyball court and plays on her college (Salisbury University) club team. Ashlyn is a part of Younglife, Fellowship of Christian Athletes, and studies community health. She may also have a future in educating young people about living with diabetes.

How has diabetes positively impacted your life?

Diabetes has positively impacted my life because it has made me become so responsible at such a young age. At only eight years old, I was counting carbs, applying ratios/correction formulas, and even giving myself my own insulin injections. Diabetes has also given me such a different perspective on everyday life. While living with such a critical disease, it has enabled me to decipher what in life is actually important. When I was diagnosed, I went into DKA and fought for my life in the ICU at Nemours AI DuPont Children's Hospital. After going through such an experience and knowing how it could happen again, it has made me live life day by day and enjoy every moment.

If you could tell someone newly diagnosed something you've learned living with T1, what would it be?

You cannot beat yourself up while living with this disease. You can do everything possible to keep your blood sugar under control, yet you still can't always control it. That's the thing about type 1; you can manage it, but so many things affect your body and your blood sugar, and everyone is affected differently. Everything from exercise, to sleep, to the weather, to stress, messes with my blood sugar levels, so I have learned that I cannot get upset every time I am faced with difficulties with this disease.

How has type 1 given you composure? Please explain a specific story.

Diabetes has made me very composed. There have been many occasions where I am on the brink of losing consciousness but must remain calm. For example, I was in New York City just the other day. It was a fun day, but exhausting. On the way home, we stopped to get food, and I even gave myself less insulin since we had been walking around all day. Suddenly, I felt dizzy, so I checked my continuous glucose monitor. I was in the 80s and rapidly dropping. Although I wasn't that low, I knew my body, and I knew it was coming. After two more readings, I was below 40 and still rapidly dropping. We were on a highway at 1:00 in the morning, could not find any exits, and I had already drunk all the soda I had brought. I very easily could have freaked out, but I remained calm. I had never been more sure that I was going to pass out. We finally made it to a gas station, and everything ended up being okay, but of course, part of me was worried that it wouldn't be. This is another example of just how unpredictable this disease can be, and composure is one of the many characteristics that diabetes has helped me obtain. Overall, I am thankful that I live with this disease, and I believe that God is going to bring good out of it.

Discipline

dis·ci·pline | \ ˈdi-sǝ-plǝn \ : *control gained by enforcing obedience or order : orderly or prescribed conduct or pattern of behavior : SELF-CONTROL (Merriam-Webster 2020)*

Discipline is a term that's often seen in the wrong light. Many think that discipline means being boring and unexciting, moving through life doing the same thing every day. While it's true that disciplined people often like to follow routines, this can be extremely important to keep them moving forward in life. This is not at all a bad thing; it's just how their brain works. The same is true for us living with type 1, as it forces us to follow routines day in and day out.

Some of my personal routines include taking a long-acting insulin shot every morning and changing my continuous glucose monitor every ten days. Other type 1s have to change out their insulin pump every three days; others must give long-acting insulin shots at night and in the morning, not to mention all the routines that come along with eating and dosing for meals and any non-diabetes routines like school, work, exercise, etc. People with T1D need routines to stay healthy. To follow those routines, we must stay disciplined every day, or else we directly feel the consequences. We indirectly learn to stay on-track just by doing what we must do to stay alive every day.

Aside from just discipline of the body, we build an immense discipline of the mind as well. This can often be seen in our nutritional choices. As type 1s, we know that it's probably a better idea to eat complex carbohydrates such as rice or grains instead of the simple carbohydrates in something like a cupcake. While I'm sure that cupcakes taste great, we know we won't be feeling too hot later when our blood sugar levels are skyrocketing. So, we choose the complex carbs (most of the time) as we know it's better for our health and our blood sugar levels. However, for the times when we do pick the cupcake, we have the discipline to count the correct number of carbs, give our insulin, and wait a grueling fifteen minutes for that insulin to start doing its work in our body before we eat. Which, by the way, makes the food taste so much better when that much prep work goes into eating it.

This learned discipline can be applied to literally any other area of life as well, especially school and work, because nobody likes the undisciplined kid in school who is rowdy and obnoxious or the un-disciplined co-worker who can't seem to finish his projects before the deadline. This is one of those traits that forces young people with type 1 to mature even faster. Most children I know can barely remember to put pants on every morning, let alone have the discipline to remember to give their morning shot of insulin. Pants *and* insulin? Kids with type 1 are pretty amazing, right?

Spotlight: Nicole E.

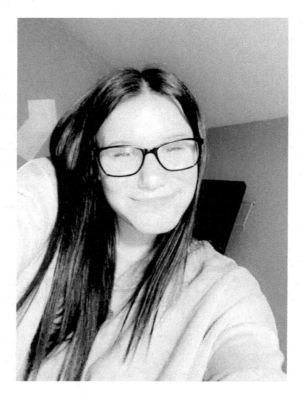

Bio

Nicole is sixteen years old and was diagnosed with type 1 at age four. Nicole is the type of person who seems to always be laughing and makes everyone around her do the same. Come to think of it, I don't think I've ever seen her without a smile on her face. Nicole also loves to sing and is in her school choir and pep club.

How has diabetes positively impacted your life?

Sure, it makes it hard sometimes to be around people and not be able to always do everything they are because of high or low blood sugar. But that forces you to slow down and appreciate life. Plus, I've made great friends because of it.

If you could tell someone newly diagnosed something you've learned living with T1, what would it be?

Do not let it change who you are. It may get hard, but you are never alone in it. People may not always understand, but know it's going to be okay.

How has type 1 made you disciplined? Please explain a specific story.

I have to remember to stay with my routines, keep all my supplies with me, and be patient when my blood sugar levels are high/low to wait for them to return to a good number. One time, I forgot my insulin at home and went to my friend's house almost an hour away. Unfortunately, I had a very high blood sugar level, got sick, and had no insulin, blood testing kit, or anything I needed. I went home, and even after I had taken my insulin, it took me till the next day to even come down to a healthy level. I had to be patient and wait for insulin to work so I wouldn't feel bad anymore. That taught me to never forget my insulin and to stay disciplined.

Accuracy

ac·cu·ra·cy | \ ˈa-kyə-rə-sē , ˈa-k(ə-)rə- \ : *freedom from mistake or error : CORRECTNESS : conformity to truth or to a standard or model : EXACTNESS (Merriam-Webster 2020)*

Being accurate is something that lots of us could care less about. For most kids, it doesn't matter exactly how much cereal they eat in the morning. Forgot to pack the right amount of snacks for your pickup basketball game? No worries, you'll remember next time. Unfortunately, it's not this simple for us type 1s. If I didn't know the number of carbs I ate for breakfast, it would throw off my blood sugars for the rest of my day, affecting how I feel and perform. If I were to forget to bring enough snacks for a basketball game and have a hypoglycemic episode (dangerously low blood sugar), I could pass out on the court. And nobody wants to have the job of strategically injecting cake frosting into a big, pale, sweaty guy's mouth to hopefully bring him back to consciousness.

Being accurate is important in so many aspects of life. Something as simple as using the correct amount of flour in the cake you're baking can make or break the results. Putting the right amount of gas in your car today can determine how your morning commute goes tomorrow. The same is true for living with diabetes, but with a lot more risk involved. When dealing with dosing insulin, the difference of a unit can literally be the difference between life and death, and that's no joke.

Learning to be accurate takes time, diligence, and effort. Having diabetes, we are forced to be accurate with everything from exact measurements of food to the syringes we fill every day. This constant need for exactness in our treatment carries over anywhere in life. Super accurate young people with diabetes make for amazingly capable adults who can tackle any challenge life tosses their way.

Spotlight: Justin K.

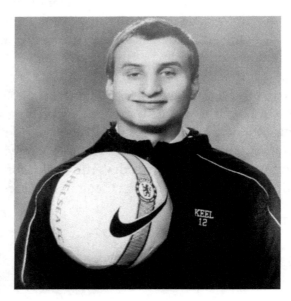

Bio

Justin is eighteen years old and was diagnosed with diabetes at age seven. Justin is hilarious, has made me laugh way harder than I'd like to admit, and is wicked good at *Cards Against Humanity*. He also excels at soccer and plays on his school team. Justin has a passion for sports cars and one day hopes to drive his dream car: a Lamborghini Aventador.

How has diabetes positively impacted your life?

Diabetes has positively impacted my life by giving me new friends who are more like family, making me more responsible, and giving me hope that one day they'll find a cure.

If you could tell someone newly diagnosed something you've learned living with T1, what would it be?

I would tell a newly diagnosed type 1 diabetic that taking care of yourself is more important than it seems. You don't want to wait until you have a bunch of life-changing complications to do it, so take preventative measures. Also, getting a good A1C blood test result is like a challenge, and I love pushing myself to succeed at it. Think of it as a challenge instead of something you're forced to do.

How has type 1 made you more accurate? Please explain a specific story.

Diabetes has made me more accurate in life in multiple ways. In one way, it has enabled me to be more precise with how my body is feeling. For example, when my blood sugar is very low, I feel like I'm going to pass out. When it's high, I feel like I'm going to throw up. This ability extends beyond diabetes. I'm also an athlete, so this allows me to sense when I'm going to get hurt before I do. It's pretty much like a superpower. The other way it makes me more accurate is in a problem solving/math sort of way. As a diabetic, I have to give a certain amount of insulin for however many carbs I eat. The problem is that not all foods come in containers with nutrition labels on them. When we aren't given a carb amount, we're forced to guess. Just like in sports, the more you do it, the better you get at it. My family loves to go out to eat, so I must guess my carbs more than I'd like to. This helps my estimations and guesses in the real world, too. I can't tell you how many times I've guessed how long it takes to get from here to there and have actually been right. Yet again, it's like a superpower. I mean yeah, diabetes sucks sometimes, but can you accurately tell me how many carbs are in a cup of rigatoni? I didn't think so.

Maturity

ma·ture | \ mə-ˈchu̇r , -ˈchər also -ˈtu̇r , -ˈtyu̇r \ : *based on slow, careful consideration (Merriam-Webster 2020)*

Maturity seems to have different meanings to different people. To me, someone who is mature can see the importance and seriousness of a situation and act on it accordingly. This doesn't mean being serious all the time; that would just make life pretty boring, right? I know this firsthand as I'm pretty much the least serious person I know.

Maturity is often associated with age, where older individuals are seen as being wiser. I can confidently confirm this is not always the case. I've met some adults who can barely hold their composure around a skinned knee, yet I've watched six-year-old children who can insert insulin pumps with harpoon-sized needles into their skin without a second thought.

Given the intensive nature of diabetes care, kids living with the disease are forced to grow up quickly. Being responsible for your own livelihood every hour of every day is important. One wrong push of a button on an insulin pump could send you to the hospital in a coma within a matter of hours.

Although extremes like this are rare, they do happen. This just goes to show the importance of seeing the seriousness in every treatment decision and being able to act accordingly. The fact that kids with type 1 learn such impressive maturity from such a young age helps mitigate most issues and leave them happy, healthy, and thriving for life ahead.

Spotlight: Savana M.

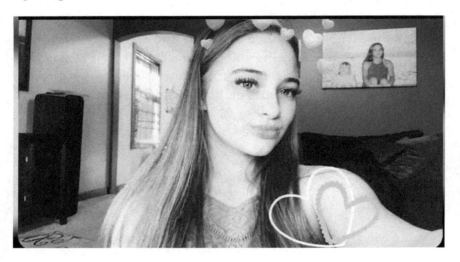

Bio

Savana is seventeen years old and was diagnosed with diabetes at age eight. She is a high school student and loves cheerleading. In addition to regular schooling, she is also completing a pre-nursing program at a local technical school, making her one of the hardest workers I know. She'll be headed to nursing school soon after graduation.

How has diabetes positively impacted your life?

Making amazing connections, friendships, and getting great resources from diabetes camp.

If you could tell someone newly diagnosed something you've learned living with T1, what would it be?

Try to take the best care of yourself but don't feel like you're terrible when you go low or high, it happens, and you can't be perfect. What's most important is how long your numbers stay high or low. Also, always carry juice, and be very patient with your body!

How has type 1 made you mature? Please explain a specific story.

Diabetes has made me mature from a young age because I've always had to put more thought into what and how much I eat, along with the math that goes into dosing myself. Being a kid and giving yourself needles every day just to stay alive is a huge responsibility.

Organization

or·ga·ni·za·tion | \ ˌȯr-gə-nə-ˈzā-shən , ˌȯrg-nə- \ : *the act or process of organizing or of being organized (Merriam–Webster 2020)*

I pride myself on being a pretty organized dude. What other twenty-one-year-old do you know who uses file folders on a consistent basis? I'm not obsessed with neatness, but I function better when everything is in its place. I fully attribute this to living with diabetes.

The heaps of medication and supplies it takes to tackle diabetes can get ridiculous at times. Syringes, lancets, BG meters, CGM, CGM insertion devices, CGM transmitters, insulin pens, pen needles, alcohol wipes, skin-tac wipes, pump reservoirs, pump sites, pump tubing, insulin vials—just to name a few. I have an entire closet dedicated to diabetes stuff. Judging by the sheer amount of junk we always need to have in stock, it makes sense why organization is key to success with type 1.

Make sure to keep all your supplies stocked and clean, and it's happy days. Forgetting to order something or running out earlier than you thought is panic-inducing, to say the least. Remember, this is life-saving medication we are dealing with. Having extra meds on hand is a must because you truly never know. You must also always be prepared with extra-low blood-sugar treatment whenever you leave the house. It may be a little excessive, but in my school backpack, I carry a tube of glucose tablets, a mini-squeeze bottle of maple syrup, and usually a piece of fruit. My preparation, organization, and neatness have steered me clear of some sticky situations.

Even something as simple as measuring your food before you eat it and neatly arranging it all while you count the carbohydrates can play a big role in your ability to organize. Same with packing up your diabetes bag, or "betus bag," as my friends like to call it. Make sure you pack enough of everything, including insulin, snacks, blood glucose meter, test strips—the whole nine yards. Dealing with these things day in and day out leads to neat and tidy kids who grow up to be neat and tidy adults who can tackle any challenge life gives them.

Spotlight: Ryan S.

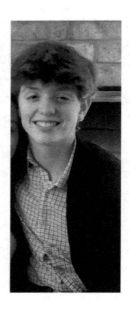

Bio

Ryan is fifteen years old and was diagnosed with diabetes at age five, on the day after Thanksgiving. He enjoys riding his bike, playing many different sports, lifting weights, and hanging out with his buddies. Ryan's a funny dude who can put a smile on anyone's face.

How has diabetes positively impacted your life?

Having type 1 diabetes has been a struggle, but the life-long lessons I have learned outweigh all the negatives. I have built character and learned to be brave and resilient. I have also made many friendships that continue to grow each year.

If you could tell someone newly diagnosed something you've learned living with T1, what would it be?

I would tell them that being responsible with your diabetes treatment is always worth it. As long as you are careful, it will be okay! Also, have fun with it and meet new people in the process.

How has type 1 made you organized? Please explain a specific story.

Being a person with type 1 diabetes has made me very responsible and organized. I must always monitor and keep track of my diabetes because I know how important it is. Being organized with all my supplies and with my time and schedule is key to good treatment. Along with that, I have been taught not to make excuses and that I am always accountable for what happens to me.

Patience

pa·tience | \ ˈpā-shən(t)s \ : *the capacity, habit, or fact of being patient (Merriam-Webster 2020)*

Patience is something I always struggled with as a kid. I was never really one to sit still, and I hated waiting in lines. I was the one asking, "Are we there yet?" in the back of the minivan and don't even get me started on when my parents ran into a friend at the grocery store. But luckily, life with type 1 has taught me to be a bit more patient and be more comfortable waiting.

Type 1 requires strong patience, plain and simple. Insulin takes time to work once it's injected. Often, uninvited high blood sugar will come along (possibly from the heaps of ice cream you ate earlier), and you'll have to endure hours of waiting just for it to come back down to normal. (The cookie dough was definitely worth it, though!)

Another classic example is all the equipment failures that come along with type 1. Diabetes medical technology is amazing, but everything good comes with its flaws, and things don't always work as they should, which leads to headaches and blood sugar spikes.

This all means that I didn't gain my newfound patience overnight. It took lots of tantrums about high blood sugar levels and failed insulin pumps to get to where I am today. And I'm not in any way perfect, I still get impatient when it comes to dumb little things sometimes. But the fact that I've been able to calmly endure the fifteen-hour flight from the USA to Australia twice says something about the patience I've gained.

Kids with T1D become superstars when it comes to patience. This translates to the real world because, as cliché as it is, good things come to those who wait, whether it's waiting patiently for their blood sugar to level off, waiting in lines, dealing with others, or anything else in life. Yet another life skill sharpened by life with type 1.

Spotlight: Katie C.

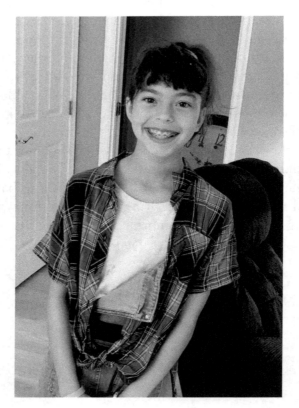

Bio

Katie is ten years old and was diagnosed with type 1 at age eight. She loves to stay active and never lets diabetes stand in her way. She plays travel basketball, runs 5Ks with her mom, and loves hanging out with her family and her dog, Archie. Katie is also quite the artist; she loves painting and building with Legos.

How has diabetes positively impacted your life?

It has made me feel healthier. I've learned about the benefits of good nutrition. I've learned to make sure everyone fits in and doesn't feel different.

If you could tell someone newly diagnosed something you've learned living with T1, what would it be?

Get a CGM. Fewer finger pricks. Don't be afraid of shots and finger pricks, insulin helps you to be healthy!

How has type 1 made you patient? Please explain a specific story.

It's given me patience and a new outlook on friends. I might be a little different, but I don't want anyone else to feel different. I always make sure I'm kind to everyone!

Gratitude

grat·i·tude | \ ˈgra-tə-ˌtüd , -ˌtyüd \ : *the state of being grateful :*
THANKFULNESS (Merriam-Webster 2020)

As I mentioned earlier in this book, I'm beyond thankful for the fact that I have type 1 diabetes. Yet, I seem to get quite the shocked response when I tell this to others. Thankful? For a horrible, life-threatening condition? How is that even possible? Living with a chronic condition like this really teaches you to slow down and appreciate everything life has given you, including diabetes.

Life with diabetes naturally comes along with some pretty tough days, but that's nothing to get discouraged about. It only means that we can be that much more grateful for the great days; those days where our blood sugar level stays in range, where our pump insertions don't hurt, and where we remember all of our supplies. It even helps us to appreciate the not so great days, seeing the good in everything. Blood sugar levels high today? Well, it could be much higher. Insulin pump failed at home today? Well, it could've happened at school. Diabetes has been a huge influence on my overall mindset, that there will always be a positive that comes out of everything in life, no matter how dark it may seem.

I'm not the only type 1 I know who lives with this outlook on life. People with type 1 have true gratitude as they appreciate the delicacy of their lives and appreciate anything and everything they are given. They can be more grateful for their health and lives overall as they see the consequences when things don't go as planned. Something simple I've noticed is that kids with T1D are exceptional at saying please and thank you. This alone says a lot about their character and the appreciation for life that they'll carry for years to come.

Spotlight: Grace H.

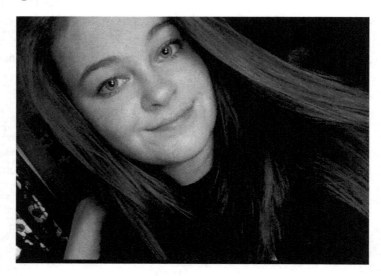

Bio

Grace is sixteen years old and was diagnosed with diabetes at age five. She radiates kindness and loves to stay moving, playing field hockey, unified bowling, and bocce. She enjoys spending time with her friends and family, especially playing sports outside with her brothers. Grace is also an NHS member and part of the FLIP club. Her favorite activity is playing with her two dogs and two cats.

How has diabetes positively impacted your life?

Diabetes has impacted my life positively in several ways. It has given me a tremendous support system as well as a strong mind. I have learned to overcome several issues that have occurred along the way, but I made it through, and now I brush off negative comments. It has also given me the power to change people's minds about diabetes. There are several stereotypes surrounding it, but I feel like I'm helping to break those barriers, and more people are starting to understand how it truly affects people and that it's not something to joke about. I have also gained many friends, even a second family. I personally think that is very special, and it's something that I'm lucky to have.

If you could tell someone newly diagnosed something you've learned living with T1, what would it be?

If you think your life is over because you were diagnosed with diabetes, trust me, it's not. Yes, you will have to completely change your life around. Yes, you will face hardships. And yes, you will feel like you don't want this disease, and you will feel upset that it was given to you. But you just need to keep pushing through and do what you need to do to make sure you are as healthy as can be. Always take care of yourself. Every diabetic at one point or another has felt like they want to give up, or that they don't care. But you need to take care of yourself. It may only seem like rebellion now, but it will greatly affect you later in life. If you choose not to take care of yourself, you're only hurting yourself more and causing severe damage. Don't let what people say affect you. Do not give them the power or satisfaction of hurting you. Show them you are strong and that their words don't hurt you. You'll be so much happier when you realize they have no power over you.

How has type 1 taught you gratitude? Please explain a specific story.

Diabetes has given me so many reasons to have gratitude. Firstly, it has made me extremely grateful for my mom. She has been my biggest supporter since day one, and I honestly don't know if I could have done it without her. She helped me learn how to manage my diabetes and helped me through all the bad times I've had because of my disease. She is so selfless that she would rather have me need what I have, rather than need her. She has made many sacrifices for me and my diabetes; I couldn't be more grateful for her. I know we may argue about how I manage myself, but I know it's because she loves me and only wants the best for me. I am very thankful to have a mom like her, I know many diabetics don't, and it truly makes me feel so lucky that I have a mom who is also diabetic so we can go through everything together. We're like a team, building off of each other and helping each other through this.

I am also grateful to my other family members, like my dad and my brothers. They always help me when I need it, and they don't treat me any differently because of my diabetes. It may be a small thing, but it really helps me get through this, knowing that my family is behind me through it all.

Diabetes has also grown my gratitude for my friends. I have friends who always check in on me, as well as friends who carry around extra candy in case I go low. My best friend even has glucose tabs in her nightstand if I ever need them in an emergency. I feel so thankful that they also don't change the way they treat me because of my diabetes. It makes me feel good that they don't look at me like I'm different.

I am also very grateful for camp. Camp has given me a place where I feel safe because everyone is like me. I don't feel like I stand out. I'm surrounded by people who feel in similar ways that I do. I think it's very important that every child with diabetes has a place where they can feel safe, and I am so thankful that I have mine.

I have a great sense of gratitude for my medication. I am fortunate enough to be able to afford my medication and the supplies I need to manage my disease. A lot of diabetics can't afford their insulin, which can lead to becoming seriously ill. Even if I don't show it, I am so very grateful for my supplies and insulin to keep me healthy.

But I think I gained my greatest sense of gratitude from becoming stronger. When I was younger, I faced a lot of hardships relating to diabetes. From being diagnosed so young, to dealing with all the school bullies, I have learned that this disease does not define me. Yes, it's a very big aspect of my life, but it is not what defines me. I know my worth, and I know I am so much more than this disease and their words.

When I was in kindergarten, just after being diagnosed, there was a boy in my class who bullied me ruthlessly. He spread rumors about diabetes being a plague that would kill you if you came near me, would say things to me, and always had a very negative attitude toward me. I would be scared to go to school because I was worried about what they were going to say to me. I would cry for my mom all the time, and I would sit in the counselor's office to help myself calm down.

Because of his actions, I had very few friends until third grade. Only then did some of the kids start accepting me. In middle school, I was scared the same thing was going to happen, so I tried to hide it as much as possible. But later in middle school, I realized after telling some of my friends and having them accept it that I was going to be okay. There were a few bumps in the road with some people, but I made it through. And now, I'm proud to show that I'm a diabetic. I'm grateful that I had those experiences, even if they weren't the best situation for me. They helped me accept myself and my situation, and I am extremely grateful. They made me have a strong mind, and it taught me that their words don't matter, only me taking care of myself does. And for that, I am truly grateful.

Forethought

fore·thought | \ ˈfȯr-ˌthȯt \ : *a thinking or planning out in advance : consideration for the future (Merriam-Webster 2020)*

Forethought is just a fancy word for thinking about your future. If you haven't noticed, most young kids aren't really the greatest planners. Kids are experts at "going with the flow," which is something most of us adults could serve to be a bit better at. However, living with type 1, your future is something you must consider every day with every single treatment decision you make.

The better your blood sugar levels are now, the fewer complications you'll have in the future. The thought of horrific health issues later in life is a bit scary, but it's a good incentive to make sure you're always doing your best when counting carbs, giving insulin, and treating low/high blood sugar levels. I'm not sure about you, but when I hear that I could possibly lose my foot if I have poor blood sugar control, that makes me very careful with my treatment. I'm not always a fan of scare tactics to get people to do things, but in this case, it works well.

Many of the kids with type 1 who I've been lucky enough to meet are some of the most driven people I know. Full of passion, whether it's for a hobby, sport, or anything else, they work hard to do what they love. They consider the future, not only with their diabetes but with everything else in life. I know lots of kids with type 1 who already have their hearts set on going into medicine when they're older to give back to the medical community that they've grown to know so well. I also know lots of grown adults with type 1 who have done just that and are some of the most amazing health professionals I've had the pleasure of working with.

Foresight isn't something that comes naturally, and being conscious of your future isn't easy, but people with type 1 almost always do an amazing job of it.

Spotlight: Mackenzie "Mack" L.

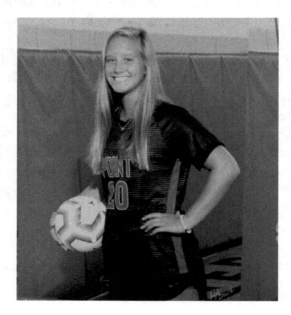

Bio

Mack is sixteen years old and was diagnosed with diabetes at age ten. She is a multi-sport athlete who plays soccer, basketball, and tennis, yet somehow still finds the time to be dual-enrolled in high school and community college. She also interns at a local elementary school as she's looking to become a teacher. Mack is a wonderful singer and exhibits admirable compassion toward everyone around her.

How has diabetes positively impacted your life?

Diabetes has given me the opportunity to meet new people, have a healthier lifestyle, and get better at mental math. Every day brings new struggles with this disease, but my goal is to always come out stronger. It's not something I've "gotten used to," as most people think, but it's something I've accepted and made the best of and have not let it affect what I love to do.

If you could tell someone newly diagnosed something you've learned living with T1, what would it be?

Since being diagnosed with T1, I've learned that I'm never alone. There is always someone who has gone through the same obstacles I may come across. It's also very important to find a support system of not only your family and friends but people who are also T1 because they understand what you're going through and can always help. Going to a diabetes camp and making friends who also have T1 was probably one of the most helpful things I've done for myself and one of the best experiences I've ever had.

How has type 1 given you forethought? Please explain a specific story.

Being a type one diabetic for six years now has given me a lot of forethought. I am always thinking about what my life will be like when I'm an adult and how diabetes will affect it. As bad as it may sound because I'm only sixteen, I've considered how my blood sugars and health will be affected if I drink alcohol—when I'm twenty-one, of course. I've thought a lot about the financial side of being diabetic as well. I am very blessed with two wonderful parents who can do a lot for me, and I've thought about how my life will change when I'm an adult and no longer living with them. Having T1 has caused me to think about my future earlier than most kids and be fully prepared for life as an adult with type one diabetes.

Self-Awareness

self-aware·ness | \ ˌself-ə-ˈwer-nəs \ : *an awareness of one's own personality or individuality (Merriam-Webster 2020)*

Self-awareness and mindfulness are fancy buzzwords that people like to throw around. They're often associated with yoga or meditation, and they mean being aware of yourself, both body and mind. They also mean being in touch with how you feel. Luckily, you don't have to sit outside cross-legged under a tree to work on your self-awareness. Living with type 1 diabetes will help you get in touch with your body unlike anything else.

Every time my blood sugar begins to drop, I begin to feel a bit groggy, my eyes seem to move a bit slower, it's harder for me to focus, and I feel weak, tired, and have barely any energy. When my blood sugars go too high, I feel thirsty, a bit nauseous, and irritable. Very irritable. (You can ask my mom about that one.) Everyone I know with type 1 feels a bit different when their blood sugars are changing. Some may even get a seizure when they go too low—pretty scary stuff. With diabetes, you must be very in touch with the way you feel, because your life depends on it! The more in touch with how I'm feeling, the better I can treat my always changing blood-sugar levels.

My own self-awareness has saved my life more than a few times. I've been in the middle of intense lacrosse games and been feeling a little bit off, so after subbing out and checking my sugar levels, I found they were dangerously low. A few more minutes on the field, and I would have been face down in the turf. You can tell how important it is to be in touch with how you feel at all times.

Kids with type 1 aren't shy about it either. They know their bodies better than anyone and aren't afraid to put their health first. This makes for mindful kids who end up being very self-aware adults, ready to tackle life ahead with an impressive ability to stay in touch with their own minds and bodies.

Spotlight: Ben C.

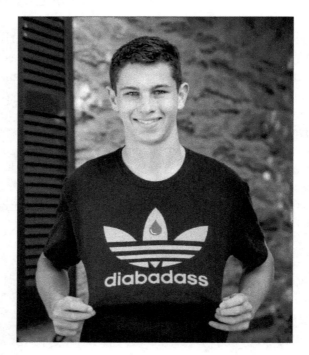

Bio

Ben is seventeen years old and was diagnosed with diabetes at age twelve. He participates in a variety of activities, including varsity soccer and track, and his soccer team won the state championship in 2018. I can tell you from personal experience that Ben is quite the beast on the soccer field. I've been scored-on by him more than a few times during our matches at diabetes camp. He also works as a math tutor, helping children from 2nd through 12th grade with many different topics. He volunteers at his church in many roles, ranging from dishwashing for weekly fish fries or being a religious education aid. He also is a member of the Ambassador Program at his school, where he meets with children who are struggling academically or socially and helps provide them with the support they need to be successful.

How has diabetes positively impacted your life?

Diabetes has positively impacted my life primarily by making me more disciplined and responsible with how I manage my health. The amount of planning and self-awareness that I need to commit to a routine to keep my blood sugar level in range makes me more mature than a lot of kids my age. With this maturity also came independence, as I quickly learned how to read my insulin pump reports and perform all my injections in case I went somewhere without my parents and had to fend for myself. Diabetes has also allowed me to develop relationships with people that I would never have met otherwise. Ever since the first fall after I was diagnosed, my family has consistently attended the JDRF OneWalk in Philadelphia, which exposed me to a tight-knit community of Type 1 Diabetics that embraced me with open arms. The amount of encouragement and support that I received from those people about how diabetes would not prevent me from doing anything I wanted to do has inspired me to work twice as hard as those around me, which I know will pay off in the long run. In addition to the JDRF OneWalk, I have attended a summer camp for diabetics known as Camp Possibilities for the past four years, where I made friends with teenagers my age who were in the same situation as me. Having the opportunity to not only hear multiple perspectives about how to manage your disease from people in your situation but to also mentor kids younger than you who are new to the disease has made me very open-minded and sensitive to the unique problems each individual camper experiences on a daily basis. So even though diabetes is relentless, it has blessed me with a support system and lifelong values to ensure that I can move confidently into a future filled with hope and possibility.

If you could tell someone newly diagnosed something you've learned living with T1, what would it be?

Something I've learned living with T1D is that it's okay to not be perfect all the time. I learned this very early on with T1D because after the honeymoon phase where I was taking minimal insulin and still maintaining tight control over my blood sugar levels, I suddenly experienced spikes after meals that I had never seen before. Initially, I thought that it was a poor reflection on me that I couldn't keep my sugar in range for as long as I wanted it to, which made me a "bad" diabetic. However, I had to swallow my pride, and not only view my glucose readings as information, but also every day as an experiment rather than a grade of my performance. You are not going to have perfect control all the time, so there is no use stressing about it. My doctors simply advised me to do the best that I could using my CGM and glucose meter to keep track of my general trends and make adjustments as necessary.

How has type 1 given you self-awareness? Please explain a specific story.

Type 1 diabetes has made me more self-aware because I exhibit specific physical symptoms when I'm both high and low, which requires me to be in tune with the way I'm feeling to ensure that I can keep my blood sugar levels in check.

I never imagined that it would take an episode with moderate ketones to remind me of just how important self-awareness is, but I, unfortunately, found myself in that position during my sophomore soccer season. Following an intense match where adrenaline had spiked my blood sugar, I went to the concession stand to grab a hamburger before I had to be a ball boy for the varsity match. At that moment, I should've realized that eating a hamburger while I was already high and not dosing was a horrible idea, but I was paranoid about the effects of the adrenaline wearing off and me not having enough energy to run up and down the sideline for eighty minutes. At halftime of that game, I noticed all the telltale symptoms of me being high: thirst, nausea, and a pounding headache. However, I was also caught up by the game, and fear of dropping low still lingered in the back of my mind, so I continued to leave my pump disconnected.

With about five minutes left to go in the game, the nausea had only gotten worse, and my mouth was drier than the desert, so I texted my mom to be ready with the car for when the game was over. After the ref blew the final whistle, I mustered what little energy I had to run to her car, as it was too late for a pump bolus; I desperately needed a shot from my insulin pen.

Not even a mile from my house, after trying to suppress my nausea for what seemed like an eternity, I barely rolled the window down in time before projectile vomiting all over the side of her van. I will never forget the bewildered look on my dad's face when we pulled into our driveway with vomit all over the passenger side door; my pale, ghastly face told him all that he needed to know. Within minutes, I was sprawled out on the couch with my blanket and Powerade, sick as a dog, as my mom frantically explained the situation to the emergency diabetes hotline at Children's National Hospital in Washington. They advised that my mom give me shots of both Levemir and Humalog, as a blood sugar over 400 with moderate ketones would not resolve itself quickly.

Fortunately for me, by the next morning, my blood sugar had returned to a reasonable level, but that harrowing experience made it apparent that I should've listened to my body at that moment by dosing before it was too late. From that moment forward, I vowed to carry my pump supplies with me wherever I went, and I recently added the continuous glucose monitor to my regimen to more accurately monitor patterns of highs and lows throughout the day.

Levity

/ˈlevədē/ /ˈlɛvədi/ : *Humor or frivolity, especially the treatment of a serious matter with humor (Oxford 2020)*

This word may be a bit foreign to you; I know it was for me, Yet, it sums up most everyone I know living with type 1 perfectly. In our world today, there are a lot of serious things happening. Between politics, climate change, crime, corruption, and all the other depressing things you see in the news, it's easy to feel disheartened. Pile living with a chronic disease on top of that, and things get even rougher. But what's one thing that can help us all to smile, laugh, and enjoy the good in life just a bit more? Humor. There's a reason that people turn to stand-up comedians, romantic comedies, and shows like NBC's *The Office* in tough times. Humor takes the negativity of the world and flips it around, taking something once cried over, and turning it into something to belly laugh over. Levity just means staying lighthearted through rough times and being able to use humor as a wonderful tool for positivity.

People with type 1 have levity unlike any other group of people on earth. It takes a special kind of human to, rather than dwell on their circumstances, constantly make jokes about it. This is especially true when it comes to something as serious as type 1 diabetes. It makes the scary stuff—giving shots, counting carbs, and treating low blood sugars—that much easier when there's some laughter behind it.

People with type 1 have an uncanny ability to downplay their quite-serious life-threatening disease with jokes and laughter among others with and without type 1. I know I did for almost my entire life, and it's part of what shaped my positive mindset toward my condition today.

At diabetes camp, for example, it's essentially a week of joking around with other amazing T1Ds. It's an absolute free for all, and where the best jokes truly come out, probably due to the fact that other type 1s are the only people who will understand most of them. Jokes about never changing your lancets, CGMs peeling off, and high blood sugar levels don't usually get a great laugh among my non-diabetic friends. However, when I am with anyone who's non-diabetic, me making light of my daily struggles with diabetes puts them at ease. Making them laugh about it means making them feel comfortable. This could mean being more comfortable around me and all my bionic medical devices or more comfortable about diabetes in general without worry that something they say about my type 1 may offend me. (But I promise, *nothing* offends me.)

Learning levity through having type 1 makes for some hilarious, fun-loving people who never take themselves too seriously. This makes all the hardships we go through (diabetes or non-diabetes related) that much more bearable and actually pretty funny, in my opinion.

Spotlight: Tommy W.

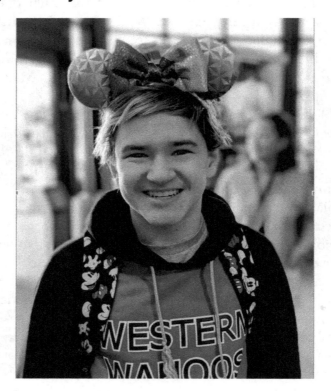

Bio

Tommy is fifteen years old and was diagnosed with diabetes at age seven (on Easter, actually). He loves playing video games with his buddies, baking, and cooking. More recently, he's been learning to build himself a new computer—from scratch. Pretty cool, huh? You can always count on Tommy for a contagious smile and for the latest and greatest type 1 meme to brighten your day.

How has diabetes positively impacted your life?

Diabetes has impacted my life greatly. I've made new friends, my life has improved, and most importantly, I am able to go to an amazing camp for diabetics like me.

If you could tell someone newly diagnosed something you've learned living with T1, what would it be?

Take help! I know how much it might kill you to do so, but asking for help is okay. The people who offer it are there for you. They can give pretty good advice, and they are willing to give it to you. And remember, orange glucose tabs are the worst!

How has type 1 given you levity? Please explain a specific story.

You know that old saying that laughter is the best medicine? Well, that's not entirely true. Insulin is the best, but laughter is a close second. Putting a smile on someone's face feels almost as good as coming back from a low blood sugar level. While getting diagnosed in the hospital, I learned that I needed to make the best out of all of this. And so I have. If you treat a lot of things with humor and levity, you'll find that life will be so much more fun.

Pride

\ ˈprīd \ : *the quality or state of being proud such as : inordinate self-esteem : a reasonable or justifiable self-respect (Merriam–Webster 2020)*

My diabetes is probably the most important thing in my life, and it will become the same for you. I tend to talk about my diabetes a lot, so I've gotten the "we get it, your diabetic" joke from my buddies plenty of times. I love it, and it always gets a good laugh, yet I thought about it, and I'm sure some kids hear that complaint more often and in a more hostile way from others… Honestly, there's nothing else in my life that I've spent more time on than my diabetes. Not a hobby, not school, not work, not anything, and it's the same for all of us long time type 1s. It makes sense to want to talk about something that literally takes over every single day of your life.

It's quite common to see very young people with type 1 being shy and timid about their diabetes, such as hiding their insulin pump or only checking their blood sugar level away from other kids. Trust me, I was there once, and I totally get it. But something magical happens once we hit a certain age; we begin to fill with a strong sense of pride for our condition and the struggles it's taken us through. I can attest to this as I've lived it and know an amazing community of type 1s who have, too. We now flaunt our insulin pumps and continuous glucose monitors like they are scars of the battles we've overcome. If you told an eight-year-old, shy, timid me that in a few years I would be writing an entire book about diabetes, I never would've believed you.

You could hide it from others in fear of feeling weird, or you could be proud and take diabetes for what it is. A tough challenge that's amazingly impressive to overcome. I promise people will look at you with amazement when you do amazing things in life, not pity and judgment. An example I like to use is my time playing high school lacrosse. My team and coaches obviously knew quite well that I had type 1, and I made sure of that. It ended up that my coaches gave me the nickname "Juice-box" since I was always treating low blood sugar levels with juice. I loved it, and the team loved it too. When you are proud of the challenges you face, others will return that energy right back in a positive way.

You must be your own advocate. Be proud of what you've been through and what you'll go through. I encourage you to talk about your condition every chance you have. It will give others more respect for you than you ever imagined. Remember, if it's okay for people to endlessly go on and on about what reality TV show they watched last night, it's perfectly okay to talk about the life-threatening disease that you live with every second of every day.

Spotlight: Logan D.

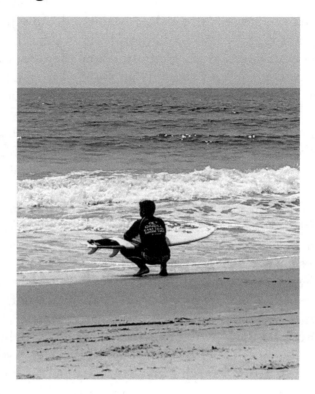

Bio

Logan is thirteen years old and was diagnosed with type 1 at age twelve. He's only been battling type 1 for a year, but rather than letting it shut him down, he's done the opposite. Logan continues to stay active playing lacrosse and football and spends his free time hunting and fishing. He also is a competitive surfer and spends his weekends traveling around the east coast beaches. Shaka, dude!

How has diabetes positively impacted your life?

The biggest way type 1 diabetes has positively impacted my life is I'm more mindful of what I eat. I don't eat as many snacks with unhealthy carbs as I used to.

If you could tell someone newly diagnosed something you've learned living with T1, what would it be?

It isn't as bad as it seems. What I mean by this is that you may think at first that you are restricted in the things you can do, but you really have just as much freedom. It's all about planning.

How has type 1 given you pride? Please explain a specific story.

Being a T1D has given me pride by being able to connect with other athletes who are T1Ds on a different level. For instance, Mark Andrews, who is a tight end for the Baltimore Ravens (my team). Also, I have been able to meet my friend Ally, who is a fellow lacrosse player.

Adaptability

/əˌdæp.təˈbɪl.ə.t̬i/ : *An ability or willingness to change in order to suit different conditions (Cambridge 2020)*

nyone living with type 1 will tell you, things never really seem to go as planned when treating your diabetes. You can be extremely calculated with your treatment, and seemingly "do everything right" yet things will not always work out as we would like them too. This simple fact forces us to become adaptable, willing to change and able to truly "go with the flow."

Being adaptable means that when things don't go as planned, you are able to remain calm and do what you need to do to fix them to get back on track. In other words, diabetes treatment isn't black and white. It's full of blue feelings, sickly green faces and red blood stained jeans. Your body changes, your environment changes and your health changes... So, you ADAPT!

My favorite example of this is quite relatable for anyone who uses an insulin pump. These pumps are amazing pieces of technology, yet the pump and its accompanying supplies sometimes don't work as they should. This spells trouble for us T1D's, as it literally means that the device that should be pumping the life saving medication into our skin, is no longer doing so. Unless you live with, or have lived with a Type 1, it's hard to understand the frustration that this brings about. Non-diabetics have never had to deal with the feverish act of dropping everything they're doing and switching out their pancreas… When our pumps decide not to work correctly, we must be able to adapt to the situation. I've changed out my insulin pump site in some weird locations, the middle of the forest included.

Throughout all these issues we face on a regular basis, we learn to face our challenges, and adapt accordingly. Life outside of T1D isn't black and white either, so once you become great at adjusting to new or challenging situations, you'll be that much more equipped to handle anything life throws your way. Being adaptable with your diabetes teaches you to be willing to change and to think on your feet when life throws you a curveball, which it DEFINITELY will.

Spotlight: Brandon M

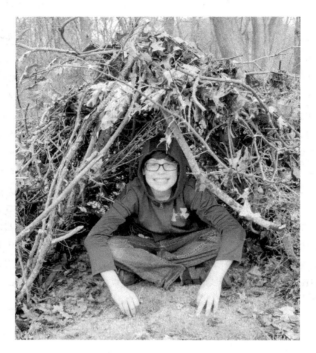

Bio

Brandon is 12 years old and was diagnosed with Type 1 just two weeks before his first birthday. He loves fishing, heading to the beach and playing all kinds of sports, especially baseball, basketball, and football. He also enjoys drawing and painting. Brandon LOVES to learn about history, figure out how things work and can often be found taking things apart and putting them back together. Needless to say, he is a well rounded little dude who doesn't let type 1 stand in the way of all of his awesome hobbies.

How has diabetes positively impacted your life?

My life has been positively impacted because of diabetes in many ways. God has opened a door to talk to others about the good news gospel. When my blood sugar goes low, I get to eat food. Diabetes has helped me to learn healthy habits. Meeting with Nutritionists who teach me healthier habits and how to live a happier life. I get to make friends that also have Diabetes and go to camp where we get to learn from each other. Diabetes has allowed be to become more responsible. I make sure that I am on a good schedule from eating and correcting my blood sugars, to getting good sleep, to changing and updating my diabetic technology.

If you could tell someone newly diagnosed something you've learned living with T1 what would it be?

In the beginning coping with Diabetes is not easy, be patient with yourself. It gets better the more you learn. There are so many people and resources to help you through this transition. The hardest thing is to not be overwhelmed. Take one day and one goal at a time. Set small manageable goals for yourself. For example, try to have good blood sugars for one day and celebrate when you do accomplish this goal. Try to focus on the good things that happen with your diabetes!

How has type 1 made you adaptable? Please explain a specific story.

One Sunday morning at church my blood sugar was a little high. When I walked into church someone had brought donuts. I really wanted a donut even though I knew it wasn't a good idea. I ate the donut anyway and felt extremely sick. So I sat on the porch with my Mom and we talked about better ways to deal with this kind of situation in the future. I figured out that I need to be smart about my choices. That day I decided to become adaptable to be able to enjoy the things that may seem normal. I decided in the future I will wait until my blood sugar is in a good range to have a treat like this. I also need to make sure to accurately cover for carb correction. This was the first time that I realized in all areas of my life I can be adaptable and because of this skill I can still have a normal life.

Community

com·mu·ni·ty | \ kə-ˈmyü-nə-tē \ : *a unified body of individuals : the people with common interests living in a particular area : a group of people with a common characteristic or interest living together within a larger society (Merriam-Webster 2020)*

If you haven't noticed, there was a commonality between many of the answers from the children and young adults interviewed for this book, aside from the fact that they are pretty good at handling needles. Many of them mentioned the amazing friends and like-minded people they've met from living with type 1. Almost everyone I know who lives with type 1 would say that the T1D community is one of the most amazing on the planet and is arguably the biggest positive of life with this disease.

We are a community filled with people fighting similar battles, so naturally, we all have a lot in common. Yet, we are all different in our own ways and have so much to give to the world. There's a special bond between two people with type 1 that's indescribable as we know how tough it can be fighting this beast of a disease with grace and resilience every day. It brings people together in an amazing way. Some of my best friends also have type 1, and I wouldn't have it any other way.

For many of us, we wouldn't be where we are without our diabetes community; I sure wouldn't. It's what guided me into my passion for health and inspired me to write this book in the first place. More importantly, it provides a support net for the millions of us living with T1D, which I've witnessed firsthand. When a fellow type 1 is having any sort of issue, whether that be finding a place to live, paying for medical supplies, finding a doctor, or anything else, their friends are waiting there with open arms, ready to help in any way. We're also a kind and supportive bunch. Lots of older people who I know that spent many years living with type 1 now spend much of their free time giving back to this community that has given them so much. This includes time volunteering, fundraising, and even running non-profit camps for children with T1D. If I had one piece of advice on how to get involved with your type 1 community, it would be to go to camp! As lots of the type 1 warriors have said in their spotlights, there's nothing that brings us together like a week in the woods with other like-minded people with T1D.

If I had to choose one word to describe the diabetes community, it would be "selfless." That's pretty remarkable given the fact that diabetes treatment involves constantly being in check with yourself and how you're feeling. I think that alone says a lot about this amazing group of people, a group that I'm blessed to be a part of.

For this chapter on community, I've chosen to spotlight two amazing gentlemen whom I've been lucky enough to work with. They both are directors of camps for kids with type 1 and have positively affected lots of lives, including my own.

Spotlight 1: John B.

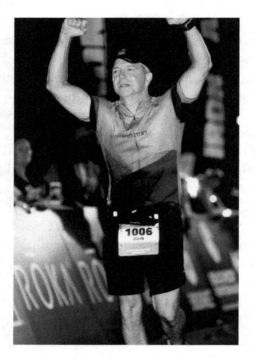

Bio

John was diagnosed when he was thirty years old and has had type 1 for twenty years. His technical profession is in marketing and writing, where he has been able to help many people write and publish books, produce educational conferences, and launch numerous businesses and podcasts. A few years after his diagnosis, he cultivated an interest in endurance sports. He began participating in triathlons fifteen years ago and has finished dozens of triathlons, marathons, and three Ironman events. He is also an amateur carpenter and often takes on projects that are "a bit over his head" (his words, not mine). John's one of the most inspirational, passionate, and helpful people I've been lucky enough to work with, and his love for the type 1 community has shown itself in admirable ways in my time working alongside him.

What is your personal relationship with diabetes?

I was diagnosed with type 1 twenty years ago when I was twenty. It was a bit unique as I didn't fit the demographic for type 1. I was older, not overweight, and somewhat active. Since then, I have noticed a trend of more people getting diagnosed with type 1 as adults.

Relationship is a good term to describe my life with type 1. We fight, we learn, I invest in it both financially and emotionally, it has punished me and rewarded me—it is like a family member. I have chosen to immerse myself in it to get the best understanding I can and to take as much control of it as possible. Like a family member, I don't always like it, and it can really piss me off, but it is a big part of me and will be for the rest of my life.

I make a choice every day that I will move forward on this journey with type 1 and make a concerted effort to learn from it. I can truly say that it has paid off. What I have learned from this journey is not limited to type 1 and has greatly exceeded anything I could have imagined.

Tell me about the camp you created. Mission, goals, activities, etc.

Being committed to learning from type 1 led me to become involved with Diabetes DESTINY. DESTINY (which stands for Diabetes Exercise Together in Network with You) is a camp that teaches kids how to be more active while managing type 1. It's in its tenth year and brings kids together with great counselors and role models with type 1 to share strategies and tips for managing blood sugar levels during intense activity.

DESTINY brings campers to a beautiful location in Maryland where they can do all kinds of activities like zip lines, kayaking, rock climbing, running, basketball, hiking, etc. while surrounded by a team of successful type 1 athletes and a full medical staff. What is amazing about DESTINY is that it takes away the fear kids might have of what can happen to their blood sugar levels when they are participating in sports or playing and shows them how to optimize their performance and improve their overall health. It also gives parents who are apprehensive about managing their child's diabetes a controlled, safe environment for their kids to learn management skills and independence.

I am currently the director, but I started out as a counselor. My goal is to get back to being just a counselor and build DESTINY into an organization that can grow and help more and more people. It is really pretty selfish for me. I love learning from the kids, and the groups of role models/counselors/volunteers are an amazing network that has really allowed me to discover great new things about type 1 that I would have never learned without them.

How has diabetes positively impacted your life?

As a writer, I am constantly working with forms and parameters. An article must be 1,000 words, this email message has to sell this product, this book has to include quizzes, a poem may have to follow certain rules. While it may be somewhat counterintuitive, those forms can inspire great creativity. Trying to hit a certain number of syllables in a haiku will make you consider words you never thought of. Getting an article down to the word count forces efficiency in your communication. Selling something in an email makes you visualize the perspective of your audience.

Diabetes, for me, has been the ultimate form. The more I learn about it, the more I understand its parameters. Trying to exist and excel within those parameters is one of the most creative challenges I have faced.

It has given me self-discipline I never knew I could have. It has helped develop deeper, more meaningful relationships by forcing me to be a better communicator. It has scared me more than I imagined possible. It has taken people from me whom I loved. It has introduced me to amazing people I would never have met and taken me to places in the world I would never have discovered.

I surely can't completely control it, but I refuse to let it control me.

Please explain the importance of community for those of us living with type 1.

As an endurance athlete, a lot of time is spent alone. Triathlons are referred to as individual sports as opposed to team sports. This couldn't be further from the truth.

On the journey with type 1, we need to surround ourselves with good people.

Fellow type 1s:

To be blunt, there is always a risk of death with type 1. To learn how to manage it requires great caution, planning, and experience. If we blindly tried things without thought, it could be fatal. This means the cycle to learn new effective management techniques is long. If we had to do this alone, we would never discover all the skills that people with type 1 have discovered. We would grow old before we figured it out or die trying, not to mention that the effort to manage life with this disease is exhausting physically, financially, and emotionally. The opportunity to know our struggles aren't unique to us and are not our fault is a critical piece of living with type 1.

Connecting with others on the same journey and immersing ourselves in the challenge with them helps us shed the overhead of feeling isolated. As we talk and communicate with other people managing type 1, it becomes more of a focus for us and allows us to see solutions we wouldn't have otherwise seen. This is a key part of why I feel being involved in DESTINY is selfish. When I spend day and night with the campers and volunteers, type 1 is an absolute focus. I learn new tips, find out about new technology, validate the feelings I have been struggling with, and discover new ideas.

Family and friends:

The impact our journey with type 1 has on the people close to us is immense. Learning to understand that impact can be transformative. When I was diagnosed, all my efforts were focused on keeping my type 1 to myself and not letting it impact anyone around me. I didn't talk about it, hid everything, and tried to not show symptoms of being low or high. There were a handful of people who were truly interested in my type 1 and my management and refused to let me share what was going on.

My wife really helped me realize that, while I was sure I was able to hide everything to keep it from impacting anyone around me, everyone knew. In fact, hiding it just made it worse. Over time, I learned how to communicate what was going on, teach those around me about type 1, and listen to the feedback they gave me. Having a CGM was a huge part of communicating. It is great to have others see our numbers, but it adds a new level to communication.

I have to make a conscious effort to be proactive in my communication. If I have a low, I must let my wife know that I have treated it so that she doesn't worry. The upside is that, when she has the context of what I was doing and what I used to treat the low, she is able to help troubleshoot and spot patterns.

For kids, working toward independence is significantly more complex with type 1. Communication is the key. The last thing a teenager wants is a helicopter parent, but they need that help to learn the skills to manage type 1 on their own. Finding that balance of how to communicate not only helps them manage better but gives them great relationship skills that they will use throughout their life.

The Diabetes-verse:

The world of type 1—from charities like JDRF and the ADA to the grassroots groups and camps to the device and pharma companies—are all an amazing ecosystem. I would like to believe that, not unlike NASA's space missions, the discoveries that the diabetes community is making will reach far beyond just managing our disease. And the environment that surrounds our community is vibrant and unique. People active in the community are more analytical, more empathetic, more driven than any other segment of society I have seen. Just look at what we have mobilized to achieve! What other group around a chronic illness has built such a robust medical device DIY community? The journey to define what life looks like with type 1 and to find a cure has created a society of exceptional individuals and will make the world a better place.

Spotlight: Jeff D.

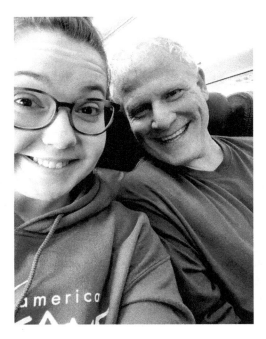

Bio

Jeff is the director of Camp Possibilities, a camp in MD for children battling diabetes. Jeff may be the most selfless and kind individual I know and has brought so much joy, growth, and learning to everyone who attends camp, myself included. Outside of camp, he loves to read and do yoga.

What's your personal relationship with type 1 diabetes?

I am not living with T1D; however, I have come to know many children and adults as a diabetes camp director since 2004. I've come to appreciate the complexity, difficulty, and ever-present nature of T1D, knowing that those living with the condition never, ever have a break. I have difficulties in life and so can relate to the persistence a condition demands, but in my estimation, there is no other condition that requires such ongoing diligence. It seems to demand the entirety of one's being—attention, emotional and mental strength and fortitude, patience, perseverance, intelligence, resourcefulness, ingenuity, and more—to live well. This includes children.

How has diabetes positively impacted your life?

I've met the most empathetic, caring, kind, mature, thoughtful, considerate, appreciative, and warm children and adults—particularly children, as that's been my relationship with diabetes. They're just amazing.

Tell me about the camp you created for kids with Type 1.

All we want to do is help, and that's how we approach camp. Hopefully, camp provides a basis for a community to form, one where others understand you and your challenges and support each other without judgment. This can be important for someone for any aspect of their well-being!

A Special Type 1 Spotlight

Mwebaza Simonpeter

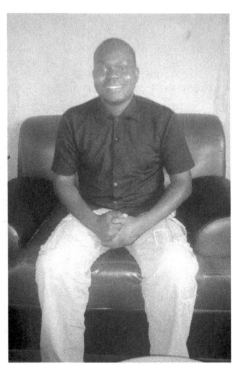

T his amazing type 1 warrior introduced himself to me on a T1D Facebook group all the way from Africa. He had heard about this book and wanted to share his story, search for some guidance, and shed some light on what it's like battling type 1 in his home country. This amazing individual, who's not much older than me, embodies all the traits and skills mentioned in this book and carries with him a special kind of gratitude for his condition. He is now what I would consider my Diabetes Pen Pal and a great friend. We often exchange recipes, photographs, stories, and messages of hope and guidance with each other. He has even taught me some of his native language. Yoga Noi Aka! Hello! This just shows the true power of the T1D community, crossing borders and changing lives everywhere on earth. Mwebaza has an extremely bright future ahead of him, and we should all aspire to see life and its challenges through the same lens that he does.

1. At what age were you diagnosed with diabetes? How old are you now?

I was diagnosed at the age of seventeen in 2013, and I'm currently twenty-four years old.

2. Tell me about where you (and your family) are from.

My family and I come from Osupa village in Pallisa district. Pallisa district is located in the eastern region of Uganda, and this is where you find my ancestral home. We are Ateso speaking people, a language that I fluently speak. I currently stay near the capital, Kampala. My people are predominantly peasants (farmers) and depend on subsistence agriculture for survival. We feed on millet flour, cassava, potatoes, rice, beans, cowpeas, and sorghum. It's important to note that most of these staple foods have a high carb content and strongly affect blood sugar levels. It's very difficult to have well-controlled glucose levels in the blood when eating such foods, and it's what the diabetics here depend on. The place here is flat land and swampy with some places full of inselbergs (an isolated hill or mountain rising abruptly from a plain). Our natives keep domestic animals that include cows, goats, sheep, chicken, turkeys, and ducks for beef, eggs, and milk. These are also sold on a small scale for income, which is usually below a dollar.

3. Tell me about some of the cool stuff you do. Interests, jobs, hobbies, etc.

I love making friends, especially those who live with type 1 diabetes. I do enjoy taking long-distance walks and hiking. I'm interested in conversations about diabetes, especially technology that we don't have here and adopted in Africa. These may include pumps, CGM machines, etc. I am always curious, and I research about new inventions in the developed world, especially those diabetes-related. I also like helping the poor since I did social work as my profession.

4. Tell me about your healthcare system in your home country. What kind of insulin treatment is typically used? What's it like getting insulin?

The healthcare system in Uganda is lacking a lot and much needs to be improved upon as compared to developed countries like America. Uganda lacks government-funded, specialized hospitals, and relies on one national hospital along with a few regional and district hospitals. A few Ugandans who have money opt for privatized medical care offered in small specialist clinics. These are usually people who work for government and corporate organizations who can afford medical insurance. Uganda has a few diabetologists, and they usually work in private clinics and are hardly accessed by the less privileged.

In Uganda, people with T1D who can afford insulin pens use Lantus and Novorapid, and those from low-income families like me use injections and purchase vials of insulin that includes Mixtard, Insulatard, and Actrapid. Insulin is usually hard to access, especially for us from low-income families. In the pharmacies, insulin like Insulatard and Actrapid costs 40,000 Uganda shillings, which is an equivalent of 10.80 USD, making it hard since most families with T1D children are poverty-stricken and earn less due to the demands of a diabetic life.

5. What is the type 1 diabetes community like where you are? Do you have other people with type 1 in your area?

People living with diabetes in Uganda face a lot of challenges, especially financial problems. To add to that, they face a challenge of stigma as the community fails to relate and accept the issue of diabetes in children. The community perceives diabetes type 1 as a curse, misfortune, and something that results from witchcraft or being bewitched, and diabetes, in general, is only perceived to be a disease for the old and rich but not children.

Some children diagnosed with type 1 diabetes fail to cope and accept the condition and pass away. Some usually go into burn out, neglect self-care and medication, and this could be attributed to weakness in parental support as well as the absence of reliable medical help. Some T1Ds die due to a lack of ability to afford insulin, and this should be mitigated. I do have a few diabetic friends, and one lives near me. Others live far from where I am, and there are a lot of children and young adults living with diabetes in different parts of the country, and the numbers grow every day.

6. How has diabetes positively impacted your life?

Diabetes has made me make a few friends, especially those with diabetes. It has inspired me to work a little harder to achieve my goals in life like every other person that lives. It pushed me to achieve goals at school attaining a Bachelor of Social Work and Social Administration of Makerere University, the third-best university on the African continent. Also, living with diabetes has trained me to become a resilient person having the ability to cope with diabetes in a resource-inadequate setting like Africa.

7. If you could tell someone who is newly diagnosed something you've learned living with T1, what would it be?

I have learned that dealing with daily pricks and injections is part of me, and a newly diagnosed person should do the same.

9. What is one message about diabetes that you would like the readers to take with them on their journey?

The reader should reflect on the difficulties in insulin acquisition faced by T1D warriors in Uganda and Africa in general, to advocate for a reduction in insulin prices and shipping of better and improved insulins used elsewhere in the developed world and the US. They should also engage in relief organizations and individuals to assist the less privileged diabetics elsewhere in the world.

Final thoughts

Through the process of writing this book and hearing from some amazing people, I've finally come to understand that, no matter where you are in life, whether it's at your lowest low or your highest high, it simply does not dictate your happiness. It's all reliant on your mindset and your attitude.

As someone with Type 1, you could look at your diagnosis as something that makes you weird and get mad about the fact that you aren't "normal." Come to think of it, what is "normal?" Nobody is truly normal; we all have things about us that make us unique. For some people, it may be the fact that one of their eyes is green and one is blue. For some, it may be that they have a lonely freckle on the left side of their nose. It just so happens that, for you, it's that you have type 1 diabetes, and that's okay.

So with that, I urge you to take this diagnosis as what it really is, the biggest challenge you'll ever face. Look at every single treatment decision as a chance to take your health into your own hands. Look at your blood sugar reading as a blessing, to be able to have a number to help guide your eating and exercise habits. Look at all the other amazing people who you can get to know that face the same challenges you do. Look at all the amazing skills you just read about that you'll have the chance to master.

You could easily dwell on the fact that you've been diagnosed with a chronic illness, or you could rejoice in the fact that you're an amazingly stronger person because of it. Spending your time sulking won't change anything, I promise. What will change your life is you tackling this condition with determination, knowing that you'll come out the other side better than you were before.

Remember to always:

- See every obstacle as a challenge to overcome
- Focus on what diabetes will give you rather than what it will take
- Don't let your condition define you; let it inspire you

For those of us living with type 1, coming to the realization that your situation won't change, so your attitude must, is the key to success and happiness. Facing your diagnosis with unforgiving optimism will allow you to far exceed your expectations of life ahead, making you stronger and more resilient than you ever imagined. Just wait until you have the chance to look back on all you've accomplished and be able to say, "Wow, all these things I've done are pretty incredible, but I did it all while battling type 1 every single day." Now that is truly incredible.

You'll have lots of people and things to thank for your success in life, but the biggest will *positively be type 1.*

Follow-up

Thank you so much for reading, I hope you enjoyed it.
Liked the book?

1. Please give it a rating on Amazon, it would mean the world!

2. Post about it on social media with the hashtag #Positivelytype1
    and follow me at:
    -   Instagram: Type1onthemove
    -   Facebook: Type 1 on the Move

3. Visit my website for more diabetes/holistic health content
    and to reach out to me directly:
    -   Type1onthemove.com

4. Fill out this short survey about the book! (Scan the code for
    access)

Works Cited

"Accuracy." *Merriam-Webster.com*. Merriam-Webster, 2020. Web. 19 May 2020.

"Adaptability." *Dictionary.cambridge.org*. Cambridge, 2020. Web. 19 May 2020.

"Community." *Merriam-Webster.com*. Merriam-Webster, 2020. Web. 19 May 2020.

"Composure." *Merriam-Webster.com*. Merriam-Webster, 2020. Web. 19 May 2020.

"Discipline." *Merriam-Webster.com*. Merriam-Webster, 2020. Web. 19 May 2020.

"Empathy." *Merriam-Webster.com*. Merriam-Webster, 2020. Web. 19 May 2020.

"Forethought." *Merriam-Webster.com*. Merriam-Webster, 2020. Web. 19 May 2020.

"Gratitude." *Merriam-Webster.com*. Merriam-Webster, 2020. Web. 19 May 2020.

"Hardworking." *Merriam-Webster.com*. Merriam-Webster, 2020. Web. 19 May 2020.

"Independence." *Merriam-Webster.com*. Merriam-Webster, 2020. Web. 19 May 2020.

"Levity." *Oxford Dictionary*, www.lexico.com/en/definition/levity. Accessed 19 May 2020.

"Mature." *Merriam-Webster.com*. Merriam-Webster, 2020. Web. 19 May 2020.

"Motivation." *Merriam-Webster.com*. Merriam-Webster, 2020. Web. 19 May 2020.

"Organization." *Merriam-Webster.com*. Merriam-Webster, 2020. Web. 19 May 2020.

"Patience." *Merriam-Webster.com*. Merriam-Webster, 2020. Web. 19 May 2020.

"Pride." *Merriam-Webster.com*. Merriam-Webster, 2020. Web. 19 May 2020.

"Problem-Solving." *Merriam-Webster.com*. Merriam-Webster, 2020. Web. 19 May 2020.

"Responsibility." *Merriam-Webster.com*. Merriam-Webster, 2020. Web. 19 May 2020.

Robinson, David. "Diabetes and Mental Health." *Canadian Journal of Diabetes*, vol. 42, no. 1, Apr. 2018, pp. 130-41, doi.org/10.1016/j.jcjd.2017.10.031. Accessed 16 Feb. 2020.

"Self-awareness." *Merriam-Webster.com*. Merriam-Webster, 2020. Web. 19 May 2020.

About the Author

When it comes to anything health and human body-related, I'm an absolute nerd. The way our bodies are woven together so perfectly to breathe, to move, to run, to walk to *exist* is nothing short of incredible. Layer that curiosity with my 17-year experience living with type 1 diabetes, and I was destined for a path of health and wellness. Having to be so in touch with my body, how I'm feeling, what I'm eating, and how I'm moving has led me to an immense appreciation for my own health and my love for helping others improves theirs.

Through meticulous nutrition and exercise strategies, along with traditional insulin treatment, I have been able to thrive with my condition while playing numerous sports, weightlifting, rock climbing, mountain biking, traveling the world, graduating college, and tackling my (too) many hobbies. I also love to spend my time learning new things, meeting new people and experiencing what this amazing world has to offer.

One of my favorite activities is spending time with others who also live with type 1, whether that be through mentoring kids with type 1 at my local hospital, being a camp counselor at various diabetes camps, or volunteering at diabetes events. It brings me true joy taking what I've spent my life learning, and sharing it with the next generation of amazing type 1s. Through all this, I've come to learn that the diabetes community is one of the most amazing groups of people on the planet, and I fully intend to commit my future to improving the lives of others with this condition type1onthemove.com.

CPSIA information can be obtained
at www.ICGtesting.com
Printed in the USA
BVHW041946160620
581683BV00010B/87